fat-burner foods

fat-burner foods

Dr Caroline M. Shreeve

hamlyn

NOTES

Standard level spoon measures are used in all recipes
1 tablespoon = one 15 ml spoon
1 teaspoon = one 5 ml spoon

Both metric and imperial measurements are given
for the recipes. Use one set of measures only, not a
mixture of both.

Ovens should be preheated to the specified
temperature. If using a fan-assisted oven, follow the
manufacturer's instructions for adjusting the time
and temperature. Grills should also be preheated.

Free-range medium eggs should be used unless
otherwise stated.

Fresh herbs should be used unless otherwise stated.
If unavailable, use dried herbs as an alternative, but
halve the quantities.

Pepper should be freshly ground unless otherwise
specified.

A few recipes include nuts and nut derivatives.
Anyone with a known nut allergy must avoid
these recipes.

FAT-BURNER FOODS is meant to be used as a
general reference and recipe book to aid weight
loss. However, you are urged to consult a health-care
professional to check whether it is a suitable weight
loss plan for you, before embarking on it.

While all reasonable care has been taken during
the preparation of this edition, neither the publisher,
editors, nor the author can accept responsibility
for any consequences arising from the use of the
information within.

First published in Great Britain in 2002 by Hamlyn
a division of Octopus Publishing Group Limited
2–4 Heron Quays
London E14 4JP

This edition published 2005

Copyright © 2002, 2005 Octopus Publishing Group Limited
Text © 2002 Dr Caroline M. Shreeve

ISBN 0 600 61287 2
EAN 9780600612872

British Library Cataloguing-in-Publication Data
A catalogue record for this book is available from
the British Library.

Printed and bound in China

10 9 8 7 6 5 4 3 2 1

Contents

Introduction

FAT FACTS

Being overweight can be an unbearable burden. How we look strongly influences how most of us feel and, while I'm sure that some people truly believe 'Big is Beautiful', for most of us being fat is the worst aspect of our lives. We long not for model figures but simply to make the best of the bodies we have.

Dieting shifts fat for as long as we maintain the effort. But the joy of reaching our target weight can banish memories of the struggle involved – and sooner or later we drop our guard and return to our old eating patterns. There is nothing surprising about this – we are creatures of habit after all, primed to seek instant gratification. Sadly, though, the backlash of frustration and despair as the weight piles back on can drive us straight into the dreaded yo-yo cycle until, scoffing and starving in turn, we end up weighing more than we did to begin with.

This has given rise to the fallacy that dieting makes you fat. It doesn't. Permanent weight loss eludes us because of the faulty methods we choose for shedding unwanted excess weight. Inevitably, as hunger pangs set in and we start to miss favourite foods, temptation becomes impossible to resist. Add low self-esteem and a secret conviction that we'll never really lose weight, and we set ourselves up to fail.

UNDERSTANDING 'OVERWEIGHT'

To lose weight, we have to use up more energy than we take in from food. For many of us, this means watching what we eat – avoiding comfort snacks and cutting down on sugary and fatty foods – and becoming more physically active. But for some very overweight people, even the strictest diet has little effect. Certainly, most studies have failed to show that obese people eat more than those of normal weight, leading researchers to look at factors other than diet to account for unmovable fat.

Recent findings blame genetic make-up for as much as 80 per cent of the variation in body fat content that exists between different people. One inherited characteristic recognized among a number of very overweight people affects their bodies' use of calories, particularly when food intake is reduced. Many frustrated dieters will have experienced the sudden cessation of weight loss that occurs when they go for hours without eating and take in fewer than a minimum number of calories over a prolonged period of time (this differs with the individual, but is around 1000–1200 calories daily for women and 1200–1500 for men).

Sensing imminent starvation and in preparation for it, the body hangs on to its fat stores and uses the energy it does derive from food for heat production, digestion and other vital functions as economically as possible. In some overweight people this specific inherited trait makes them far more sensitive than others to a reduced food intake, and their sensitive metabolism shuts down to 'tick-over' speed whenever they try to cut down on what they are eating.

We use about 60 per cent of the energy we obtain from food to keep our vital functions ticking over at rest – this is called the basal metabolic rate (BMR). The average sedentary person uses a further 20 per cent in physical activity, but, by becoming more physically active and undertaking regular exercise, both this and the BMR can be increased in normal weight and overweight people for up to 18 hours after the exercise.

Another well-publicized genetic link, discovered in 1994, was the ob-gene (obesity gene). Its protein leptin, produced in fatty tissue, affects the appetite centre in the brain, interfering with the feeling of fullness that most people experience after eating a certain amount.

DANGERS OF SURPLUS FAT

There may be genetic reasons for your difficulty in losing weight, but that does not mean that you have to join the 'Fat is Fantastic' brigade, bragging how happy you feel in your new extra-large outfit. Promoting obesity (which is defined as being 20 per cent or more over your ideal body weight) is actually dangerous. It is linked with increased risks of heart and blood vessel disorders, including high blood pressure and raised cholesterol, stroke, heart attack and deep vein thrombosis (a blood clot in a calf vein which can pass through the bloodstream to the lungs and is frequently fatal). Gall bladder disease and reflux (heartburn) are much more common in fat people. So, too, are irregular periods in women and infertility. Type II diabetes (which typically affects overweight people as mature adults), snoring and sleep apnoea (a blockage that interferes with breathing during sleep and which carries additional risks for heart attack and stroke) are also associated with being overweight.

Obesity-linked cancers are also common, affecting the large bowel, prostate, uterus, cervix, breasts and ovaries. In addition, orthopaedic problems affect overweight people more severely than lighter people, especially chronic backache and sciatica, and arthritis of the weight-bearing joints, such as the knees, ankles and the joints of the feet.

THE FAT-BURNER FOODS SOLUTION...

Sooner or later, an answer had to be found to the problem of the low energy consumption rates of the many people suffering from obesity. Like hundreds of other doctors and nutritionists, I had been researching the problem for a number of years, and coming up with only a few of the answers. Then, one magical day, a patient called Joe L. walked into my consulting room in Ingham, North Queensland, Australia and handed me a piece of paper.

'I thought you might be interested in this, doc. Me and the wife have been over in Western Australia for a family wedding and we visited cousin Bob, who is awaiting heart surgery. He had been given this diet to enable him to lose weight quickly and safely prior to undergoing a coronary bypass op. That was three months ago – he's lost 24 kilos and the doctors are very pleased with him. He's having the op next week, and he says he hasn't felt so fit for years.' Intrigued, I studied the seven-day eating plan based on two versions of a nutritious and filling soup, attributed respectively to two different hospitals in Perth, Western Australia. My attempts to discuss the diet with one or other hospital drew a blank. The cardiologists, medical and nursing staff and dieticians to whom I spoke were very cagey about it, and I was left with the impression that Joe's cousin Bob had indeed been given the prescribed diet, but that it was not intended for general use. There are several explanations and I feel that the most likely is that, while most doctors and nutritionists know that it is perfectly possible to get a lot of weight off a patient in a hurry when it is important to do so, for example prior to a life-saving operation, few if any would want publicly to endorse a diet that flies so rampantly in the face of the general advice given by the nutritional establishment.

Whatever the plan's origin, I had a number of very overweight patients on my hands, desperate to lose weight, and I decided to offer it to them to try.

Six out of seven agreed readily and I monitored their progress weekly. Meanwhile, I scrutinized the diet from the view of its fat-burning properties, since I had been researching the use of foods to increase a sluggish (i.e. obese) metabolism. It seemed to fit the bill! My willing guinea pigs were delighted with the results of the diet and claimed never to feel hungry. Further research since has led to the development of the fully fledged Fat-burner Foods Weight Loss Programme, which involves following the Rapid Fat Loss Plan for a fortnight, followed by a weight-balancing fortnight on a Stabilizer Plan, which allows a wider choice of foods and encourages the development of healthier eating habits. The complete programme works by increasing the rate at which the body burns fat, and was highly successful for 78 per cent of the people I treated.

I am confident that it can work for you, too.

Dr Caroline M. Shreeve

▶ The ingredients of success

▶ Healthy, nutritionally sound eating plan

▶ Quick, safe fat loss

▶ Easily available and filling foods

▶ Simple, adaptable menus

▶ Healthy eating for life

▶ Setting your goal

▶ Monitoring fat loss

1 Burning Body Fat

machine. When the Rapid Fat Loss Plan, consisting largely of plant foods and protein, sets this in motion, a metabolic process named ketosis kicks in. Essentially what happens is that some of the fat removed from your fat stores is incompletely burned, leading to the production of waste products called ketones. These ketones are excreted by the kidneys, and their presence in the urine (which can be detected by using a simple dip-stick test) is a sign that your body's fat-burning process has gone into fast-forward mode. Mild ketosis also acts to curb the appetite and promote a feeling of increased energy and wellbeing.

case study

Polly G., a 36-year-old housewife and mother, was 54.5 kg (120 lb) overweight when she came to see me and hating every minute of it. No diet had worked for her in the past and she despaired of any helping her in future. For Polly, The FBF Weight Loss Programme was a last resort! Unsurprisingly, her blood pressure and blood cholesterol were high and she had shown symptoms of early diabetes in her most recent (third) pregnancy. Her BMI (Body Mass Index, see page 17) was 34. She started on the Rapid Fat Loss Plan, recording her weight daily and checking in weekly for me to monitor her progress.

Polly lost an average of 3.5 kg (8 lb) a week on the Rapid Fat Loss Plan, and 1 kg (2 lb) a week on the Stabilizer Plan. After the first month (a fortnight on each plan), she had lost 9.5 kg (21 lb), and it took her just six months to lose her excess weight. Her cholesterol, blood pressure and glucose tolerance test (for diabetes) were normal, and her BMI had dropped to 24. She was playing badminton again and power walking regularly. She felt and looked ten years younger.

easily available and filling foods

There is nothing complicated about the foods you will eat while you are busy burning off fat. You will find many of your favourites listed in the menu plans and lists, and may already have some in your storecupboard and refrigerator. Fresh fruit and vegetables, meat, fish and poultry can all be combined in recipes you enjoy normally to boost the body's fat-burning capacity. You need never feel hungry on the FBF Weight Loss Programme. You are encouraged on the Rapid Fat Loss Plan to eat as many raw and lightly cooked fresh vegetables as you like, while the Stabilizer Plan utilizes a wide range of fat-burning foods, with tempting recipes and menus to help you make full use of them.

simple adaptable menus

Few of us diet in isolation. There is usually the family to cater for and, even if you live alone, there are always those packed lunches, meals out, holidays and entertaining to be taken into account.

You have to be quite single-minded on the Rapid Fat Loss Plan, but you follow it for only 14 days at a time and the Stabilizer Plan gives plenty of menu ideas to suit a variety of situations. No special cooking is necessary in order to adhere to the plan. The recipes are very easy to follow and involve relatively little weighing or measuring of ingredients. There's no calorie counting, either. The secret is knowing which foods help to burn up fat, and how and when to eat them.

healthy eating for life

For many of us, overindulgence in the past has helped pile on the weight. We know that we will have to eat differently in the future in order to maintain our new weight. The Stabilizer Plan helps you to do this by introducing a very wide range of fat-burning foods in recipes that you can continue using to maintain your target weight.

setting your goal...

Setting a specific goal when planning to shed surplus weight greatly improves your chances of success. Vague aims, such as 'I'd like to be healthier', or 'I think I'll lose a few kilos or pounds', tend to produce half-hearted efforts and poor results. Be clear in your mind about what you are going to achieve before starting on the FBF Weight Loss Programme. Write it down and put it where you will see and reread it several times a day. 'I am going to lose 6.25 kg (14 lb)' or 'I am going to go down three dress/shirt sizes' will trigger the positive thinking essential for personal growth.

Affirmations, positive statements about yourself or your intentions, are a deceptively simple aid to achieving a goal. They work by imprinting themselves upon the subconscious mind through regular repetition – saying, reading or, best of all, writing them down over and over again.

You can even record them on a suitable tape and listen to them when you are most open to their suggestive influence, for example when you are drowsy and have just woken up or you are about to fall asleep. Do whatever works best for you.

If you truly mean your affirmations and want them to come true, then they will. They do require a little discipline, but their benefits normally far outweigh the time and effort involved. If you are going to repeat them verbally, look in a mirror, smile and speak as though you mean it. Here are some ideas to get you started.

- 'I love life!'
- 'I love myself!'
- 'I'm a powerful, confident person!'
- 'I'm becoming healthy and fit!'
- 'My body is burning up fat!'
- 'I'm becoming slimmer daily!'

monitoring fat loss

You can monitor fat rather than weight reduction by using plastic skin callipers, which measure the thickness of fat in various body areas. You can also go by your Body Mass Index or BMI (see the box below). Callipers are inexpensive and available from good pharmacies. They should come with a chart indicating healthy and unhealthy fat thicknesses. However, they tend to pinch the skin and you will have to enlist help when applying them to inaccessible body areas, such as the upper back.

Probably the easiest way for you to check your body fat content is with a custom-designed body fat monitoring machine. Since body fat content is an individual issue, you will need to key in details of your height, age, sex and whether you are an athlete or do little exercise, in order to gain a really accurate measurement.

body mass index (BMI)

Obesity is defined as being 20 per cent or more above one's desirable weight range. It refers mainly to excess body fat. It is technically possible to be 'overweight' in this way without a spare tyre or love handle in sight. Since muscle is heavier than fat, body builders and athletes often weigh much more than others of the same sex, height and build. No one, though, would call them obese. Conversely, there are also apparently thin people carrying layers of surplus fat.

Body Mass Index (BMI) is a more accurate indicator of surplus body fat than kilos or pounds, although massively muscled athletes – and others who have inherited an unusually heavy build – would still be the exception to the rule. You can calculate your BMI as follows:

BMI = Weight (in kilograms)
    ÷ Height (in metres) squared
or
Weight (in pounds) x 700
    ÷ Height (in inches) squared

For example, the calculation for someone weighing 80 kg (176 lb) and 1.60 m (63 in) tall is:
BMI = 80 ÷ (1.60 x 1.60) = 31.2
    or
BMI = 176 x 700 ÷ (63 x 63) = 31.1

Body weight categories according to Body Mass Index (BMI):

CATEGORY	BMI
Underweight	under 19
Normal	20-25
Overweight	26-30
Obese	over 30

▶ **Accelerating fat-burning**

▶ **Thermogenic effect of protein**

▶ **Negative calorie foods**

▶ **Carbohydrates**

▶ **Glycaemic index**

▶ **Dietary fats**

▶ **Iodine and chromium**

▶ **Hydroxycitric acid**

▶ **Fat-burner foods**

18

2 How Fat-burner Foods Work

accelerating fat-burning

Fat-burner foods and human metabolism are highly complex issues and not yet fully understood even by nutritional scientists, so the account of them here is necessarily highly simplified and incomplete.

Certain foods and eating habits can be used to accelerate fat-burning, either directly by promoting the 'meltdown' of the body's surplus fat stores, or indirectly by fine-tuning our use of energy. Protein, for instance, significantly increases the metabolic rate (the pace at which we use food fuel), creating heat and burning many more calories than carbohydrates or fat. Negative calorie foods are those foods that use up more calories in the process of their assimilation into the body than they supply for its use. Certain sources of carbohydrates (i.e. those with the least effect on our blood sugar levels) help us to burn up the food at our disposal rather than storing it as fat. Particular food combinations, for example protein

and negative calorie foods, can be used to mobilize fatty deposits for conversion into energy, a metabolic process called ketosis (see page 14).

Depending on their nature, the fats in our diet affect – either beneficially or adversely – how we respond to insulin, a hormone produced by the pancreas. Insulin controls both the fat content of our cells and our blood sugar levels. Chromium and iodine, two vital minerals, also influence insulin and other hormones that are connected with obesity.

Lastly, certain naturally occurring substances, such as caffeine, capsaicin (found in chillies), chitin from shellfish shells, the Chinese herb Ma Huang, even aspirin (originally derived from willow bark) influence the way our bodies handle fat. Another example is hydroxycitric acid, found in the brindleberry fruit, which hinders the production of fats from carbohydrates and curbs the appetite (see page 26).

thermogenic effect of protein

While 1 gram of fat provides about 9 calories, 1 gram of carbohydrate provides about 4 calories and 1 gram of protein also provides about 4

calories. These statistics explain why most slimming diets cut down on fat. However, although fat provides, weight for weight, more than twice the energy of the other two food groups, protein has a built-in factor known as its thermogenic effect or 'specific dynamic action', which burns calories and depletes fat stores.

The very act of eating uses calories, since all food requires energy for its breakdown and digestion, absorption from the stomach and small bowel, chemical changes in the bloodstream, liver and so on, and the storage of its nutrients. But while fat has a thermogenic effect of only 0–3 per cent and carbohydrates of 5–10 per cent, protein has one of 20–30 per cent of its calorific value.

This useful thermogenic effect of food is reduced to 50–150 calories a day in obese people with a resistance to insulin (see below), so increasing the importance of protein in a fat-loss programme, and of other measures which help to sharpen the body's sensitivity to insulin.

negative calorie foods

Negative calorie foods use more calories to break down, digest and assimilate them than they supply. The surplus calories 'burn' fat in the body. For example, a portion of fruit trifle provides a total of 350 calories; 100 calories are utilized in digestion and absorption, leaving 250 calories to be added to your day's total calorie intake. However, a portion of Brussels sprouts provides 50 calories; 75 calories are utilized in digestion and absorption, thus burning 25 calories of body fat.Eating mainly negative calorie foods is said to reduce weight three times faster than fasting and to reduce body weight by an average of 0.5 kg (1 lb) a day. It is difficult to confirm these claims, but the concept of negative energy and fat-burning is at least feasible. Since many of the foods are either high-protein or low-GI carbohydrates (see page 22), they are included in the programme.

To help one's metabolism 'burn fat 24 hours a day', however, oxygen consumption must be increased, in the form of either planned aerobic exercise such as brisk walking, cycling or swimming, or specific breathing exercises (see page 118).

dietary fats

A high total fat intake also lowers insulin sensitivity. Conversely, monounsaturated fats have a beneficial effect. An Italian study conducted by G. Ricardi and reported in the *British Journal of Nutrition* in 2000, gave 162 healthy adults a diet high in either monounsaturated or saturated fat, for three months. Results showed that the former significantly improves insulin sensitivity compared with a diet high in saturated fat (fat derived from animal products). However, this beneficial effect disappears when the total fat intake accounts for more than 38 per cent of the total calories consumed.

However, trying to eliminate fat from the diet completely is unhealthy. It is a vital, life-giving nutrient and, if we don't eat as much fat as we need, our bodies make it. Nor do reduced-fat diets in themselves create weight loss. This point is illustrated in the results from a study in the US. In 1955, Americans were getting 40 per cent of their calories from fat; by 1995 the percentage had fallen to 35; in the same period the percentage of overweight adults increased from 25 per cent to 40 per cent. It seems that many people construe a low-fat diet as licence to eat as much as they want of other foods, regardless of calorie content. At the same time, all developed societies are becoming increasingly sedentary, which is another important factor.

unsaturated fats

Our main source of monounsaturated fat is olive oil, the cold-pressed extra virgin variety being the healthiest. Derived from the first pressings of ripe olives, it is crammed with nutrients undamaged by the industrial heat-processing which alters and destroys them. Omega-3 oils, polyunsaturated fats found in fish, seafood, green leafy vegetables and walnut oil, reduce unhealthy blood fats and help guard against heart attacks. Both oily fish and cold-pressed extra virgin olive oil are used extensively throughout the FBF Weight Loss Programme.

Fat will not create extra fat in your body unless you take in more calories than you use. The healthy approach is to keep your energy intake from fats below 38 per cent, cut down saturated fat and include a significant proportion of olive oil and its products and oily fish, such as sardines, mackerel, salmon and tuna, which contain the essential fatty acids.

iodine and chromium

Iodine is necessary for the normal function of the thyroid gland, which controls the BMR (basal metabolic rate) (see page 7). Iodine deficiency can result in thyroid underactivity, thereby lowering the BMR and causing an increase in weight. Losing weight when one has low levels of thyroxine – the main hormone produced by the thyroid, and which cannot be manufactured without iodine – is practically impossible without undergoing some form of medical treatment.

Whether supplemental iodine does help to speed up a sluggish BMR in the absence of a proven deficiency is a moot point. Kelp (a seaweed) is a rich source of iodine, which explains why it is often included in patent slimming formulas. Besides seaweeds, iodine is present in sea fish, seafood and sea salt.

Chromium is required by the body to help it deal with carbohydrates and dietary fats. Combined with the B vitamin nicotinic acid (niacin) and tryptophan or some other amino acid, it constitutes the glucose tolerance factor (GTF chromium), which decreases insulin resistance and drives circulating glucose into the tissues. Diets high in carbohydrates can lead to chromium deficiency; this, as well as the ageing process, impairs the body's ability to make GTF chromium, so then specific foods and supplements are required.

Chromium supplements have been used to improve blood glucose control in sufferers of both Type I diabetes (where the body lacks its own insulin) and Type II (late-onset) diabetes and have reduced their insulin and other medication requirements in some instances. Chromium also promotes the uptake of amino acids (the breakdown products of protein digestion), thereby helping to increase lean body mass (LBM) and decrease stored body fat.

Foods rich in chromium include brewer's yeast, oysters, beef, wholewheat products, potatoes and liver, all of which appear in recipes in the FBF Weight Loss Programme. However, a daily 400 micrograms (mcg) supplement of chromium picolinate is recommended as part of the Rapid Fat Loss Plan to accelerate fat-burning.

hydroxycitric acid

The rind of the brindleberry fruit is widely used in Asian cooking, as a flavouring in curries instead of limes or tamarind. According to scientific reports (in the *Journal of Biological Chemistry* in 1971 and the *American Journal of Clinical Nutrition* in 1977), the hydroxycitric acid (HCA) found in the rind can inhibit the production of cholesterol and other blood fats from dietary carbohydrates.

Dietary carbohydrates are broken down into glucose. Some is used for energy and the rest is stored as glycogen in the muscles and liver. Once the glycogen stores become full, an enzyme named ATP-citrase lyase turns any excess glucose molecules into cholesterol and fat. HCA appears to inhibit this last stage, reducing fat production by between 40 and 70 per cent for up to 12 hours after a meal. HCA also curbs the appetite, because excess glucose is no longer being turned into fatty tissue and therefore remains stored as glycogen. Glycogen stores remaining at a high level signal to the brain that energy reserves are full and no more food is required.

HCA is also thought to be the active ingredient in the juice and rind of grapefruit and possibly other citrus fruits, which have similar effects to brindleberry. Grapefruit and citrus fruits are therefore included in a fat-burning diet, while brindleberry is best taken as a dietary supplement (available from healthfood stores).

note

The list of negative calorie foods opposite is incomplete, but covers the main foods you enjoy and are used to eating. Use your judgement about others; for example since cress is included, it is fine to use similar sprouting vegetables, such as alfalfa, fenugreek, radish and mung bean sprouts. All raw or lightly cooked vegetables, fruits and nuts in their natural state, provide negative calories, while dried and canned fruits and roasted salted nuts do not.

OTHERS
Cold-pressed extra virgin olive oil and its products
Iodine-rich foods: e.g. edible seaweed such as kombu and nori; sea salt, fish and shellfish
Chromium-rich foods: e.g. brewer's yeast, beef, oysters, wholewheat products, liver and potatoes
Brindleberry and citrus fruits

Fat-burner foods

Some fat-burning foods belong in more than one class, for example negative calorie foods and low-GI, or negative calorie and protein. For simplicity's sake, the foods are grouped here under the main class to which they belong. See page 23 for low-GI foods.

FAT-BURNER PROTEIN FOODS

Lean meat: beef, pork, lamb, veal, venison, rabbit, hare, offal
Poultry: chicken, turkey, pheasant, grouse, guinea fowl
Fish: cod, haddock, plaice, sole, coley, whiting, mackerel, trout, salmon
Shellfish: scallops, shrimp, prawns, lobster, crab, scampi, cockles, mussels, winkles, whelks, abalone
Cheese: mainly low-fat cottage cheese and low-fat fromage frais. Use reduced-fat versions of hard cheeses, such as Cheddar, in moderation
Eggs
Soya products

NEGATIVE CALORIE FOODS

Vegetables: asparagus, aubergine (eggplant), beetroot, broccoli, Brussels sprouts, cabbage, carrots, cauliflower, celeriac, celery, chicory, Chinese cabbage (pak choi, bok choy), cress, dandelion leaves, endive, fennel, globe artichokes, green beans, leeks, lettuce, mangetouts (snow peas), onions, radishes, seaweed, spinach, squash, swede, tomatoes, turnips
Fruits: apples, apricots, bananas, blackberries, blackcurrants, blueberries, boysenberries, cherries, clementines, cranberries, damsons, figs, gooseberries, grapefruit, grapes, greengages, guavas, kiwi fruit, kumquat, nectarines, oranges, papaya, peaches, pears, persimmons, pineapple, plums, pomegranate, prickly pear, raspberries, redcurrants, satsumas, star fruit, strawberries, whitecurrants
Nuts: almonds, Barcelona nuts, Brazil nuts, chestnuts, coconuts, filberts, hazelnuts, macadamias, peanuts, pine nuts, pistachios, walnuts

▶ Starting the plan

▶ Charting your progress

▶ The principles

▶ Rapid Fat Loss Plan guidelines

▶ The 14-day Rapid Fat Loss Plan

▶ Recipes

3 The Fat-Burner Foods Rapid Fat Loss Plan

starting the plan

The diet is an extremely healthy one (as we saw in Chapter 2) and suitable for most people (but see below). However, I always err on the side of caution and, because I have never met you and cannot, therefore, monitor your progress, I advise you simply to check first with your own doctor. This is especially important if you suffer from any ongoing health problems, take regular medications and/or you are a teenager or over 65 years old.

After the initial fortnight on the Rapid Fat Loss Plan, the FBF Stabilizer Plan – of which there are four versions in all (see Chapters 4 and 5) – gives you a chance to acclimatize to your new weight and eat a wider range of foods. It is generally rather less demanding than the FBF Rapid Fat Loss Plan and, although most people could safely repeat the first fortnight without a break, the 28-day programme suits most slimmers best.

health check

Check with your doctor before starting the Fat-burner Foods Weight Loss Programme if you have any health concerns or are being treated for a serious or long-standing medical condition. It is also imperative for you to obtain your doctor's approval if you are under 20 or over 65 years of age. Children, adolescents and elderly people have specific nutritional needs that the Fat-burner Foods Weight Loss Programme does not undertake to meet. Your doctor will be able to tell you whether the programme is right for you.

charting your progress

There are also extremely important psychological benefits to be had from following a programme for a specific time. You can keep tabs on your progress by crossing off the days on a calendar to encourage you to keep going, and filling out the 14-day charts of your weight loss provided on pages 122–123.

The FBF Weight Loss Programme leaves nothing to chance: your need for variety in the foods you eat, your short-term goals and your personal feel-good factor are all taken into account in this plan. This is why it can help you to succeed, no matter what difficulties you may have experienced with dieting in the past.

Despite all you have read in the past about weighing yourself only weekly (or actually throwing your scales away), dieters on the FBF Weight Loss Programme should weigh themselves daily. Unexpectedly high losses on some days will sustain you over the day or so when your weight appears to get stuck – you are not failing, it's just your body and metabolism adjusting themselves to the effects of fat-burning foods.

positive indicators

✔ You have generally good health
✔ You are aged between 20 and 65
✔ You eat most common foods
✔ You do not suffer from any food allergies or only from allergies with which you can safely cope
✔ You can organize your meals around the complete Fat-burner Foods Weight Loss Programme

the principles

The FBF Rapid Fat Loss Plan provides all the essential nutrients over a seven-day period (the second week is a repeat of the first), and helps you to burn body fat mainly through the use of negative calorie foods (see page 21). Eat the Fat-burning Soup daily at mealtimes and as a snack whenever you feel peckish. Remember, you need never go hungry on the FBF Weight Loss Programme.

You will notice that the main omissions from the FBF Rapid Fat Loss Plan are of fruit and vegetables with a high sugar/starch content, and of fatty or oily meat and fish. Some of these will appear in recipes elsewhere in this book. They are excluded here because the FBF Rapid Fat Loss Plan is based upon the simplest and healthiest foods with a negative calorie content. Lean meats other than those mentioned can be eaten (see negative calorie foods list, page 27);

but 'treated' foods containing these meats, such as ham, sausages, canned and preserved meats, should be avoided for the time being.

Use organic ingredients whenever possible – you will have to use your common sense about these. Fresh organic foods are becoming more widely available and less expensive. Organic honey is now widely available – choose clear, set or honeycomb, depending on the requirements of the recipe. You can choose between white and black ground pepper, green, pink or other peppercorns as you like, unless otherwise specified by the recipe. Spices, such as chilli powder and cayenne pepper, help to speed up fat-burning. Salt is not used as an ingredient in any of these recipes; however, you can use a potassium (low-sodium) salt substitute if you dislike unsalted vegetables and other savoury dishes.

Rapid Fat Loss Plan Guidelines

DO

✔ Follow the eating plan exactly. Substitute only as suggested.

✔ Drink at least 8 large (300 ml/½ pint) glasses of plain, bottled or filtered water daily, plus herbal teas, tea and coffee, if you wish, without milk or sweetener.

✔ Remove all skin and fat from meat and poultry.

✔ Eat your Fat-burning Soup (see page 36) or snack on raw salad vegetables from the negative calorie foods list (see page 27) whenever you feel hungry.

✔ Use only the recommended dressings for salads and other dishes.

✔ Weigh yourself naked first thing every morning, after going to the toilet. Record your weight on a chart (see pages 122–123).

DON'T

✖ Drink alcohol, soft drinks, fruit juices or beverages with sugar or milk, except as indicated in the recipes.

✖ Use artificial sweeteners if you can avoid them – your taste buds will soon get used to the different taste.

✖ Buy sad-looking fruit or vegetables, or any foods past their sell-by date. The message is fresh, fresh, fresh!

✖ Be tempted by offers of snacks or other foods – this programme is for your benefit.

✖ Gulp your food. Instead, take time to savour its smell, taste and texture, chewing slowly and thoroughly.

The 14-Day Rapid Fat Loss Plan

	DAY 1 & DAY 8	DAY 2 & DAY 9	DAY 3 & DAY 10
BREAKFAST	• Mango Smoothie (page 38) or Melon and Grape Salad (page 38).	• Chilled Fat-burning Soup (page 36). • Platter of lightly cooked vegetables.	• Mango Smoothie, Melon and Grape Salad (both page 38) or mixed fruit.
LUNCH	• Fat-burning Soup (page 36). • Soft fruit: 3–4 plums, greengages or apricots, a peach or nectarine or a bunch of currants or cherries.	• Fat-burning Soup (page 36) with chicory to dunk. • Big bunch of steamed asparagus or broccoli, dressed with Farmhouse Dressing (page 80).	• Fat-burning Soup (page 36) with apple slices or chicory leaves to dunk. • Soft fruit.
DINNER	• Fat-burning Soup (page 36) with apple slices to dunk. • Fresh fruit platter – grapes, greengage or plum, sliced apple, pineapple, pear and peach, conserving as much juice as possible.	• Fat-burning Soup (page 36). • Spicy Baked Potato (page 40). • Braised Vegetables with Dill and Mustard (page 37).	• Fat-burning Soup (page 36). • Vegetable platter. • Fresh fruit salad.
NOTES	• Snacks: any fresh fruit, except bananas and tropical fruit with a high sugar content. • At least 8 large glasses of water.	• Eat lots of raw or cooked vegetables, except peas, pulses, corn, parsnips, yams, sweet potatoes. • At least 8 large glasses of water.	• Eat any fresh fruit as Day 1 and vegetables as Day 2. • At least 8 large glasses of water.

DAY 4 & DAY 11

• Milkshake made
with skimmed milk
and bananas.

• Fat-burning Soup
(page 36).
• 2 bananas.

• Fat-burning Soup
(page 36).
• 2 chopped bananas
with a sprinkling of
freshly grated
nutmeg.

• Up to 8 bananas,
1.2 litres (2 pints)
skimmed milk and
8 glasses of water.
• Expect to lose
1.75–3 kg (4–7 lb) by
day 4.

DAY 5 & DAY 12

• 125 g (4 oz) dry-
fried lean steak,
sliced tomatoes and
tomato salsa.

• Fat-burning Soup
(page 36).
• Dry-fried lean steak.
• Tomato and chicory
or cress salad with
Farmhouse Dressing
(page 80).

• Fat-burning Soup
(page 36).
• Lean steak and
tomatoes as for
breakfast or lunch.
Or, stir-fry tomatoes
without oil, with a
handful of spinach or
watercress added at
the end of cooking.

• Try to eat 300–625 g
(10–20 oz) lean steak
and 500 g (1 lb)
canned tomatoes or
6–7 fresh tomatoes.
• At least 8 large
glasses of water.

DAY 6 & DAY 13

• Dry-fried lean steak
and mushrooms.

• Fat-burning Soup
(page 36).
• Rainbow Salad
(page 80).

• Fat-burning Soup
(page 36).
• Dry-fried lean
steak.
• Primavera Stir-Fry
(page 39).

• You can choose any
vegetables you like
from the negative
calorie foods list
(page 27).
• At least 8 large
glasses of water.

DAY 7 & DAY 14

• Carrot and Celery
Juice (page 59).

• Fat-burning Soup
(page 36).
• Warm Rice Salad
with Lemon, Garlic
and Herbs
(page 41).

• Fat-burning Soup
(page 36).
• Oriental Risotto
(page 41).

• Make as much fresh
juice as you like from
produce on the
negative calorie foods
list (page 27).
• At least 8 large
glasses of water.

Fat-burning Soup

You can vary the total weight of the fresh vegetables – use 250–500 g (8 oz–1 lb) at a time and make up a fresh supply of the soup at least every two days. Keep it in the refrigerator. You can substitute one or more of the vegetables with an equal weight of any you prefer on the negative calorie foods list (see page 27). Wash all the vegetables, but do not peel them. The more finely you slice and chop them, the more quickly and evenly they will cook.

Makes 900 ml–1.2 litres (1½–2 pints)

2 bunches of spring onions or 1 large
    onion/leek, finely chopped
1 medium or ½ large cauliflower, divided into
    florets (include the green leaves) or
    2 medium or 1 large head of broccoli
125 g (4 oz) spinach or ½ small cabbage,
    chopped
1 large red, green or yellow pepper, cored,
    deseeded and chopped
6–8 celery sticks, chopped
2–3 large carrots, thinly sliced
1–2 teaspoons each crushed cumin and
    coriander seeds (optional)
1 quantity Home-made Chicken or Vegetable
    Stock (see page 37)
4–5 large ripe tomatoes, quartered or 400 g
    (13 oz) can tomatoes
juice of ½ large lemon or 1 lime
1 small handful of coriander or flat leaf
    parsley, roughly chopped
2 garlic cloves, finely chopped or
    crushed (optional)
¼–½ teaspoon cayenne pepper (optional)

1 Place all the vegetables except the tomatoes in a large saucepan with the crushed spices, if using. Add the stock and extra water, if necessary, to cover. Heat gently until nearly boiling, then add the tomatoes and the lemon or lime juice.

2 Add the herbs and garlic, if using. Season to taste with cayenne pepper, if liked.

3 Simmer the soup for 20–30 minutes, or until the vegetables are tender.

Home-made Chicken Stock

Chicken stock is simple to make and well worth the effort. The outside, coarse sticks of celery are perfect for this recipe.

Makes about 600 ml (1 pint)

1 chicken carcass or a selection of chicken bones
1 unpeeled onion, quartered
2 carrots, sliced
1 celery stick, sliced
2–3 bay leaves
1 tablespoon chopped herbs (such as parsley, thyme, rosemary, sage) or ¼–½ teaspoon dried mixed herbs
1 tablespoon (or more) jelly left over from roasting a chicken (optional)
pepper
pinch of low-sodium salt

1 Place the chicken carcass or bones in a large saucepan with the vegetables and herbs and the jelly, if using. Season with pepper and low-sodium salt.

2 Cover with water, bring to the boil and skim off the scum that rises to the surface. Reduce the heat, cover and simmer for 30–60 minutes, topping up with a little boiling water from time to time, if necessary.

3 Strain the stock and discard the vegetables and bones. The stock can be stored in the refrigerator for up to 3 days. It also freezes well.

Braised Vegetables with Dill and Mustard

For this recipe you need 500 g (1 lb) or as much as you can eat of your favourite leafy green vegetable, for example Brussels sprouts, spring greens, baby spinach or broccoli.

Serves 1

500 g (1 lb) leafy green vegetables
300 ml (½ pint) Home-made Chicken or Vegetable Stock (see left), or ½ vegetable stock cube dissolved in 300 ml (½ pint) hot water
1 teaspoon chopped dill
2 teaspoons wholegrain mustard
salt and pepper

1 Prepare the vegetables according to type while you warm the stock in a large saucepan.

2 When the stock is boiling, add the vegetables to the pan, reduce the heat and simmer for 5–10 minutes, until just crisp or tender. Transfer the vegetables to a serving plate with a slotted spoon. Stir the dill and mustard into the stock and season with salt and pepper to taste. Pour the stock over the vegetables.

variation

Make Vegetable Stock in the same way as chicken, but omit the carcass or bones and the jelly.

Melon and Grape Salad

You can use any variety of melon, except watermelon, for this salad.

Serves 1

1 large slice of melon
1 handful of black or white seedless
   grapes, halved
juice of ½ lime
1 teaspoon clear honey
1–2 mint or lemon balm sprigs, finely
   shredded

1 Cut the melon into chunks and tip into a bowl with its juice.

2 Add the grapes, lime juice, honey and herbs. Mix well and chill the salad before serving.

Mango Smoothie

Serves 1

1 large ripe mango
300 ml (½ pint) freshly squeezed
   orange juice
mint leaves, to decorate

1 Halve the mango and scoop the flesh and any juice into a food processor or blender. Add the orange juice and blend for 1 minute.

2 Pour into a glass. Add a few mint leaves to decorate and serve with a straw.

tip

To prepare a mango, hold it upright on a board. Slice the flesh from either side of the stone. Trim off the flesh still clinging to the stone. Score the flesh of the two large pieces in a diamond pattern, without cutting through the skin. Turn the skin inside out and slice the flesh away from it.

Primavera Stir-Fry

Serves 1

100–200 ml (3½–7 fl oz) Home-made
   Chicken or Vegetable Stock (see page 37)
   or water
2 rosemary sprigs
75 g (3 oz) green beans
1 small handful of broccoli florets
1 small handful of cauliflower florets
125 g (4 oz) mushrooms
6–8 cherry tomatoes, halved
3–4 spring onions, chopped
1 tablespoon balsamic vinegar
1 small handful of basil leaves, torn
   into pieces

1 Heat the stock or water with the
   rosemary sprigs in a large wok or
frying pan until it comes to the boil.

2 Meanwhile, clean and roughly chop
   the beans, broccoli, cauliflower and
mushrooms. Add to the boiling stock or
water. Cover the pan and shake gently
from time to time to ensure the vegetables
don't stick to the pan or burn.

3 Test for tenderness after 5 minutes.
   Add the cherry tomatoes, spring
onions and balsamic vinegar and cook
for 1 minute, stirring. Serve scattered with
the basil.

Spicy Baked Potato

Try to make the time to bake the potato in a hot oven, as oven-baked potatoes are much crisper and tastier than those cooked in a microwave oven.

Serves 1

1 large baking potato
15 g (½ oz) low-fat butter replacement
spicy low-calorie, 'no-added sugar' tomato
 salsa, to serve (optional)
salt and pepper

1 Wash and dry the potato then prick the skin with a sharp knife. Place directly on the shelf of a preheated oven, 200°C (400°F), Gas Mark 6, and bake for 1–1½ hours until cooked.

2 Slit the potato in half lengthways and scrape the potato flesh out of the skins. Mash with the low-fat butter replacement, salt and plenty of pepper.

3 Return the mashed potato to the skins and serve dressed with a little low-calorie, 'no-added sugar' tomato salsa, if you like.

Warm Rice Salad with Lemon, Garlic and Herbs

This recipe uses the total amount of rice allowed for Day 7 (see page 36). Make up this salad and eat half of it. Use the remainder as the basis for the Oriental Risotto (see right). Divide the broccoli into small equal-size florets to ensure they cook evenly.

Serves 1

65–75 g (2½–3 oz) brown rice
about 450 ml (¾ pint) Home-made Chicken or Vegetable Stock (see page 37)
2 carrots, grated
1 handful of broccoli florets
grated rind of ½ lemon
1 small garlic clove, chopped
1 tablespoon chopped flat leaf parsley

1 Cook the rice in the stock until tender, but with a little bite. This will take about 20 minutes, so 5 minutes before the rice is ready, stir in the grated carrot and broccoli. Meanwhile, mix together the lemon rind, garlic and parsley.

2 Drain the rice and vegetables when cooked, reserving any cooking juices for soup, and divide into 2 portions. Set one aside for use in the Oriental Risotto. Serve the remainder scattered with the lemon rind and herb mixture.

Oriental Risotto

Serves 1

leftover Warm Rice Salad with Lemon, Garlic and Herbs (see left)
50 ml (2 fl oz) clear stock or water
1 teaspoon Chinese five-spice powder
1 handful of cherry tomatoes, halved
1 handful of button or oyster mushrooms, halved
1 heaped tablespoon grated mooli
1 teaspoon seasoned rice wine vinegar
soy sauce, to taste

1 Heat the leftover rice salad gently in a little stock or water with the five-spice powder. When warmed through, stir in the tomatoes, mushrooms and grated mooli.

2 Stir well and cook gently for 2 minutes. Stir in the rice wine vinegar. Season to taste with soy sauce and serve.

▶ Stabilizer principles

▶ Buying and cooking tips

▶ Eating philosophy

▶ Basic Stabilizer Plan with guidelines,
daily allowances and Stabilizer
Plan breakfasts

▶ The 14-day Basic Stabilizer Plan

▶ Recipes

42

4 The Fat-burner Foods Basic Stabilizer Plan

basic stabilizer plan

The Basic Stabilizer Plan will suit you if you wish to keep within your normal budget and provide meals the whole family can enjoy. None of the recipes is expensive or complicated to make, relying, as they do, on ingredients you probably already have to hand in your storecupboard.

Some suggestions can be varied a little according to your personal taste and what ingredients are available. Runner beans, for instance, can be substituted for Brussels sprouts or spinach, while coley and 'rock salmon' make as tasty a fish pie as plaice, cod, haddock or whiting.

The fat-burning potential of the ingredients is mentioned in many of the recipes to help you remember this. Although the recipes provide ingredient quantities, many of them can be altered to suit your individual preferences. The most important thing is that you get used to eating sensibly and enjoyably, using and trusting your own judgement.

basic stabilizer plan guidelines

DO

✔ Follow the eating plan. You can omit a food you dislike, but be careful to replace it with a close nutritional equivalent: for example, you can use the same weight of lean pork, veal or fresh or thawed frozen white fish instead of chicken in Lemon Chicken Stir-Fry (Day 3). It's also worth comparing calorie counts when substituting foods – always read labels.

✔ Do eat your soup, or snack on vegetables from the negative calorie foods list (see page 27), whenever you feel hungry.

✔ Keep 'grazing', that is eat small meals and snacks every 3–4 hours.

✔ Drink at least 8 large (300 ml/½ pint) glasses of plain, bottled or filtered water daily, plus herbal teas, tea and coffee, if you wish, using milk from your daily allowance.

✔ Use only the recommended dressings for salads and other recipes.

✔ Continue to weigh yourself daily and record your weight.

✔ Remember your goal and the promises you have made to yourself and renew them daily.

✔ Steer clear of alcohol, soft drinks and sweeteners.

daily allowance

- Negative calorie vegetables (see page 27) – as much as you want.
- Fat-burning Soup (see page 36) – as much and as often as you like.
- Two pieces of fruit from the negative calories food list (see page 27) – this is in addition to any fruit listed in the daily menus.
- 600 ml (1 pint) skimmed milk or 300 ml (½ pint) semi-skimmed milk or 2 x 200 g (7 oz) cartons of low-fat natural or flavoured yogurt or low-fat fromage frais.
- 15 g (½ oz) low-fat butter replacement (such as one of the cholesterol-lowering spreads).

Stabilizer Plan Breakfasts

There are three options so you can vary your breakfast over the 14 days. The options are the same whichever Stabilizer Plan you choose.

BREAKFAST 1

- Small glass (150–175 ml/5–6 fl oz) of tomato or other vegetable juice, such as carrot juice or Carrot and Celery Juice (see page 59).
- 1 portion of fresh fruit (such as 1 apple or 5–6 strawberries), chopped into 200 ml (7 fl oz) low-fat natural yogurt and sprinkled with 1 dessertspoon wheatgerm.
- If still hungry: 1 slice of toasted/untoasted wholemeal bread with a little low-fat butter replacement from the daily allowance, yeast extract or reduced-sugar marmalade or jam.

BREAKFAST 2

- Small glass (150–175 ml/5–6 fl oz) of unsweetened natural fruit juice.
- 2 wholewheat cereal bisks with milk from the daily allowance.
- 1 portion of fresh fruit (such as 1 apple or orange, or 2 satsumas).
- If still hungry: 1 slice of toasted/untoasted wholemeal bread with a little low-fat butter replacement from the daily allowance, yeast extract or reduced-sugar marmalade or jam.

BREAKFAST 3

- Citrus segments and juice, for example ½ grapefruit, 1 orange, 1 small can of mandarin oranges in natural juice, mixed with 1 chopped banana and 1 dessertspoon of toasted sesame seeds.
- Scrambled egg made with 1 medium or large egg and milk from the daily allowance, on 1 slice of toasted wholemeal bread with 1 teaspoon low-fat butter replacement.

The 14-Day Basic Stabilizer Plan

	DAY 1 & DAY 8	DAY 2 & DAY 9	DAY 3 & DAY 10
BREAKFAST	• One of the three breakfast options available (page 47).	• One of the three breakfast options available (page 47).	• One of the three breakfast options available (page 47).
LUNCH	• Quick Tomato Soup (page 50). • Tuna and cress sandwich (tuna in brine, drained and mixed with cress, between 2 slices of wholemeal bread spread with low-fat butter replacement). • 1 piece of fruit if still hungry (or save for mid-afternoon snack).	• Eggs Florentine (page 51). • 1 slice of wholemeal bread (optional). • 6–8 plump presoaked dried apricots with 3–4 walnut halves or 2 Brazil nuts.	• Coleslaw with Peanuts (page 50). • 1 plain bagel • 2 peeled and sliced kiwi fruit topped with 1 tablespoon of natural low-fat yogurt and 1 dessertspoon of pumpkin seeds.
DINNER	• Creamy Fish Pie (page 54). • Spring greens or spinach. • 2–3 tablespoons low-fat yogurt ice-cream, plus chopped fresh fruit (optional).	• Spiced Beef with Apricots (page 56). • Vegetables and 1–2 boiled potatoes mashed with milk from daily allowance. • Baked Vanilla Custard (page 59).	• Lemon Chicken Stir-Fry (page 57). • 200 ml (7 fl oz) low-fat apricot yogurt mixed with 2 chopped fresh or presoaked dried apricots.

DAY 4 & DAY 11	DAY 5 & DAY 12	DAY 6 & DAY 13	DAY 7 & DAY 14
• One of the three breakfast options available (page 47).	• One of the three breakfast options available (page 47).	• One of the three breakfast options available (page 47).	• One of the three breakfast options available (page 47).
• Seafood and Tomatoes on Granary (page 52). • 1 apple.	• Spicy Lentil Soup (page 53). • Salad sandwich (optional), made using 2 slices of wholemeal bread and low-fat butter replacement from daily allowance. • 100–200 g (3½–7 oz) low-fat yogurt (optional).	• Toasted cheese sandwich (2 slices of light rye bread spread lightly with low-fat butter replacement from allowance and 50–75 g (2–3 oz) low-fat cottage cheese with chives with 2 teaspoons grated Parmesan cheese). • 3 fresh plums or greengages.	• As much fresh fruit salad as you like, using at least 1 citrus fruit (e.g. grapefruit or orange), 1 apple and/or pear, berries and soft fruits in season. Serve with 2 tablespoons low-fat cottage cheese mixed with 1 tablespoon sesame seeds, preferably toasted.
• Kidneys Courtesan with Jamaican Cabbage (page 56). • 1–2 boiled potatoes • 2–3 tablespoons chilled stewed apple, flavoured with a little cardamom.	• Salad Niçoise (page 55). • 100–200 g (3½–7 oz) low-fat fromage frais mixed with 2 peeled and chopped kiwi fruits.	• Orange Pork (page 58). • Green vegetables, such as Brussels sprouts or spinach. • 3–4 tablespoons boiled brown rice. • 1 handful of fresh cherries and 5–6 shelled almonds.	• Quick Fish Tartare (page 55). • 1–2 mashed floury potatoes. • Green beans. • 3–4 tablespoons fresh chopped fruit topped with a little low-fat natural yogurt and 1 teaspoon brown sugar. Glaze under a preheated grill until caramelized.

Quick Tomato Soup

Serves 2

350–450 ml (12–15 fl oz) Home-made
  Chicken or Vegetable Stock (see page 37)
6 tomatoes, chopped, or 400 g (13 oz) can
  chopped tomatoes
1 tablespoon sun-dried tomato paste
1 small onion, finely chopped
75–125 g (3–4 oz) leftover negative calorie
  vegetables (see page 27) that have been
  cooked without fat or oil (optional)
2 oregano or marjoram sprigs or ½ teaspoon
  dried oregano
dash of Worcestershire sauce or pinch of
  chilli powder
4 teaspoons natural yogurt and basil leaves,
  to garnish

1 Heat the home-made stock. Add the tomatoes and their juice, tomato paste, onion, leftover vegetables, if using, and oregano or marjoram.

2 Bring just to the boil, then lower the heat and simmer for 5–10 minutes, stirring occasionally. Add Worcestershire sauce or chilli powder to taste and blend lightly in a blender or food processor, if liked. Serve swirled with yogurt and scattered with basil leaves.

Coleslaw with Peanuts

The juice from the freshly grated vegetables keeps the coleslaw beautifully moist, and the onion provides a real kick, so there is no need for any dressing other than some freshly ground black pepper. However, if liked you could mix a simple dressing with 2 teaspoons olive oil, 1 teaspoon of clear honey and 1 teaspoon lemon juice.

Serves 1

75–125 g (3–4 oz) fresh cabbage heart,
  finely shredded
½–1 small onion, finely grated
1 carrot, finely grated
1 dessertspoon sultanas
50 g (2 oz) unsalted or dry roasted peanuts
black pepper

1 Mix together the cabbage, onion and carrot in a large bowl.

2 Stir in the sultanas and peanuts and season to taste with black pepper.

Eggs Florentine

The eggs provide protein while the spinach provides iron, calcium and magnesium for fat-burning, as well as offering negative calories. Use frozen spinach if fresh is unavailable.

Serves 1

100–200 g (3½–7 oz) fresh spinach
1 tablespoon water
1 teaspoon vinegar
1 large or 2 small eggs
freshly grated nutmeg
salt and pepper

1 Wash the spinach and place in a large saucepan with the water. Cover and cook over a medium heat for 1–2 minutes, until wilted. Season to taste.

2 When soft, cut through the spinach roughly with a sharp knife and transfer to a warmed serving plate.

3 Meanwhile, set a frying pan on the hob and pour in boiling water to a depth of about 2.5 cm (1 in). Keep the water at a gentle rolling boil. Add the vinegar to hold the eggs together. Crack each egg into a saucer and slip it gently into the boiling water. Cook just long enough to set the white while the yolk remains runny. Remove the poached egg with a slotted spoon and slide on to the spinach. Season with plenty of nutmeg, salt and pepper.

Seafood and Tomatoes on Granary

You should have no problem pleasing your family with today's lunch menu of cockles and winkles. Their very image harks back to a kinder, slower era when a small carton of what we now call 'seafood', bought from a fishmonger's stall at a market and eaten with bread and butter and vinegar, was a real treat. Many people today have never even tasted them.

Serves 1

125 g (4 oz) shelled or 250 g (8 oz) unshelled cooked mixed shellfish (such as winkles, whelks, cockles)
malt vinegar, to taste
pepper
TO SERVE:
1 hunk of granary bread
low-fat butter replacement, to spread
2 sun-ripened tomatoes (optional)

1 Flick off the little brown protective shields from the winkles and whelks using a cocktail stick (cockles come undefended), then delve into the interior of the shell for the delicious prize.

2 Dip the shellfish in malt vinegar and a little pepper, and eat with a hunk of fresh granary bread, spread with a scraping of low-fat butter replacement. A couple of sun-ripened tomatoes go well with this, too.

Spicy Lentil Soup

Don't be surprised when the rest of your family demand to try this extremely quick and tasty soup on smelling it! You do not have to soak red lentils before use. They can be stored in airtight jars or other containers for up to a year.

Serves 1–2

50–75 g (2–3 oz) red lentils
1 onion, very thinly sliced
1 garlic clove, crushed (optional)
350–450 ml (12–15 fl oz) Home-made
   Chicken or Vegetable Stock (see page 37)
½ teaspoon medium curry paste
lemon juice, to taste
low-fat crème fraîche and torn coriander
   leaves, to garnish

1 Rinse the lentils and place in a saucepan with the onion and garlic, if using, and the stock.

2 Bring to the boil, then reduce the heat; add the curry paste, stir and cover. The lentils and the onion take about 20 minutes to soften – top up with boiling water if the volume becomes too reduced.

3 When cooked, purée the soup in a food processor or blender and add a little lemon juice to taste. Turn into soup bowls, swirl with crème fraîche and scatter with coriander leaves.

Kidneys Courtesan with Jamaican Cabbage

This recipe is so called because the kidneys are saucy, bold and blushing – cooked to the point of pink succulence and not a jot more. If you prefer, replace the kidneys with 175 g (6 oz) skinless, boneless chicken breast.

Serves 1

2 teaspoons olive oil
1 onion, thinly sliced
2 lamb's kidneys, skinned, cored and halved
½–1 cm (¼–½ in) piece of fresh root ginger, grated or very finely sliced
dash of Worcestershire sauce
1 large handful of shredded cabbage
1 tablespoon lemon juice
white pepper and low-sodium salt substitute

1 Heat the oil in a large frying pan, then add the sliced onion and its juices. Cook, tightly covered, until soft. Add the kidneys, ginger and Worcestershire sauce and cook, covered, for 4–5 minutes over a low to medium heat.

2 Remove the kidneys from the pan with a slotted spoon, transfer to a plate and keep warm.

3 Add the cabbage and lemon juice to the pan, and cook over a low to medium heat, stirring occasionally. Add a little hot water if the cabbage seems too dry, and season with white pepper and salt substitute. Stir in the cooked kidneys and their juices and serve immediately.

Spiced Beef with Apricots

Serves 1

1 teaspoon olive oil
1 onion, thinly sliced
2–3 garlic cloves, crushed or finely chopped
1 cinnamon stick, halved
75–125 g (3–4 oz) good-quality minced lean beef or chicken
1 leek, sliced
2 apricots, peeled, pitted and chopped
1 teaspoon grated orange rind
juice of 1 orange
2 teaspoons finely chopped fresh root ginger
salt and pepper

1 Heat the olive oil in a pan. Add the onion, garlic and cinnamon and gently fry, covered, until brown.

2 Add the minced beef or chicken to the pan and cook gently, stirring constantly, for 5 minutes.

3 When the meat is brown and cooked through, add the leek, apricots, grated orange rind, orange juice and ginger. Cover, and cook for a further 8–10 minutes until all the vegetables are soft. Season to taste, remove and discard the cinnamon and serve.

tip

If you like liver, you could replace the mince with the same weight of thinly sliced lamb's liver for a meal loaded with iron, B vitamins and first-class protein.

Lemon Chicken Stir-Fry

Serves 1

1 teaspoon olive oil
1 small onion, finely sliced
1 large garlic clove, crushed or finely sliced
125 g (4 oz) skinless, boneless chicken
    breast, diced
1 dessertspoon grated lemon rind
5–6 baby corn cobs, halved diagonally
75–125 g (3–4 oz) mangetouts, diagonally
    sliced
1 tablespoon lemon juice
pinch of cumin
1 slice of toasted French bread or 3–4
    heaped tablespoons boiled brown rice,
    to serve

1 Heat the olive oil in a frying pan or
wok. Add the onion and garlic and
cook, tightly covered, until soft.

2 Add the diced chicken, lemon rind
and baby corn cobs and continue
cooking, covered, for 5 minutes. Stir in
the mangetouts, lemon juice and cumin,
cover and continue cooking for a further
5 minutes, until the chicken is cooked
right through.

3 Serve with a slice of toasted French
bread or some plain boiled brown
rice.

Orange Pork

Serves 1

125–175 g (4–6 oz) pork fillet, trimmed
   of fat
1 teaspoon grated orange rind
1 small garlic clove, crushed
crushed seeds from 4 cardamom pods
   (optional)
1 teaspoon olive oil
juice of 1 orange
1 tablespoon low-fat crème fraîche or
   fromage frais
1 handful of watercress, chopped
1 tablespoon chopped parsley
salt and pepper
TO SERVE:
brown rice
green vegetables, such as broccoli and
   mangetouts

1 Make several deep slits in the pork using a sharp knife to make pockets. Mix the orange rind, garlic, cardamom seeds, if using, and a little salt and pepper and use the mixture to fill the pockets.

2 Heat the oil in a frying pan and swirl it around to coat the base. Place the pork in the pan, cover and cook gently, turning frequently, for 10 minutes on each side until cooked through. Test by piercing the thickest piece with a knife; if the juices run clear, the pork is cooked. Remove the pork and keep warm.

3 Add the orange juice, crème fraîche or fromage frais, chopped watercress and parsley to the pan, and stir to blend with the pork juices and sediment. When heated through, pour the mixture over the pork fillet and serve with the rice and green vegetables.

Carrot and Celery Juice

This is an ideal healthy drink for breakfast if you have an electric juicer. Serve the juice as soon as it is made as some of the valuable nutrients are quickly destroyed on exposure to the air.

Serves 1

2 medium or large carrots
2 medium or large celery sticks
dash of Tabasco sauce (optional)

1 Cut the carrots and celery into large chunks and pass through a juicer. Stir in the Tabasco, if using. Serve immediately.

variation

Substitute 1 ripe green apple for the celery sticks to make a delicious carrot and apple juice.

Baked Vanilla Custard

The eggs and milk provide fat-burning protein, while the organic real vanilla extract is sheer heaven for the taste buds.

Serves 3–4

600 ml (1 pint) semi-skimmed milk
3 eggs
1 teaspoon clear honey
3–4 drops pure organic vanilla extract
freshly grated nutmeg, to taste
stewed tart fruit (such as Victoria plums or
    damsons), to serve

1 Warm the milk in a saucepan. Beat the eggs with the honey and vanilla extract in a bowl. Pour in the milk, whisking well. Strain into an ovenproof dish or 3–4 individual ramekins.

2 Place in a roasting tin containing 1 cm (½ in) cold water and bake in a preheated oven, 160°C (325°F), Gas Mark 3, for about 20 minutes, until set.

3 Serve hot, warm or cold with a little stewed tart fruit.

60

5 Three Alternative Stabilizer Plans

The 14-Day Luxury Stabilizer Plan

	DAY 1 & DAY 8	DAY 2 & DAY 9	DAY 3 & DAY 10
BREAKFAST	• One of the three breakfast options available (page 47).	• One of the three breakfast options available (page 47).	• One of the three breakfast options available (page 47).
LUNCH	• Avocado and Prawns on Rye (page 72). • 1 peach or 2 ripe dessert plums.	• Smoked Cod's Roe with Melba Toast (page 73). • 3–4 fresh apricots or 50 g (2 oz) dried apricots, soaked overnight.	• Smoked Trout and Rainbow Salad (page 80). • 1 handful of black or white grapes.
DINNER	• Fat-burner Steak Diane (page 86). • Steamed broccoli. • Small/medium baked potato topped with a little Farmhouse Dressing (page 80). • 1 large slice of fresh pineapple or 1 sliced banana topped with a little low-fat natural yogurt.	• Herb-crusted Lamb with Spring Greens (page 88). • 1 boiled potato mashed with a little skimmed milk from daily allowance. • Lemon jelly made with 300 ml (½ pint) water, served with 1 chopped apple.	• Mixed Grill (page 89). • Salad of watercress, orange and mint (page 76). • 3–4 tablespoons boiled brown rice with 1 tablespoon lemon or lime juice and 2 tablespoons chopped parsley. • Strawberries with Crème Fraiche and Grand Marnier (page 101).

DAY 4 & DAY 11	DAY 5 & DAY 12	DAY 6 & DAY 13	DAY 7 & DAY 14
• One of the three breakfast options available (page 47).	• One of the three breakfast options available (page 47).	• One of the three breakfast options available (page 47).	• One of the three breakfast options available (page 47).
• Wilted Spinach with Eggs and Herb Butter (page 83). • An astringent dessert after the rich main course, perhaps Minty Citrus Replete (page 101).	• Courgette Stuffed Mushrooms (page 84). • 1 slice of wholemeal bread. • Peppery salad of watercress, rocket and radishes (page 77). • 6 presoaked dried prunes with 10–12 macadamia nuts.	• Chicken Antipasto (page 70). • 2 kiwi fruits.	• Fresh Sardine Salad and Citrus Mint Tabbouleh (page 74). • Persimmon Cream (page 103).
• Chicken and Winter Vegetables (page 89). • 1–2 boiled potatoes. • Green vegetables such as Brussels sprouts, spinach or broccoli. • Fruit Fanfare (see page 102).	• Seafood Vermicelli with Tomato and Mushroom Sauce (page 95). • Walnut and Honey Yogurt (page 102).	• Whiting Stoker with Green Beans and Cayenne Potato (page 96). • Fresh fruit salad made with ½ grapefruit, 2–3 slices pineapple and 1 pear, and a little ground cinnamon.	• Spiced Turkey on a Bed of Potato (page 91). • Broad beans. • Traditional Baked Apple (page 103).

The 14-Day Vegetarian Stabilizer Plan

	DAY 1 & DAY 8	DAY 2 & DAY 9	DAY 3 & DAY 10
BREAKFAST	• One of the three breakfast options available (page 47).	• One of the three breakfast options available (page 47).	• One of the three breakfast options available (page 47).
LUNCH	• Celery and carrot sticks and broccoli spears served with 2 tablespoons low-calorie mayonnaise, for dipping. • 2–3 crispbreads. • 1 whole fruit such as an apple or orange.	• Cottage Cheese Salsa on Toast (page 72). • 2–3 mandarins.	• Viva Tomatoes on Toast (page 75). • 15–20 black or white grapes.
DINNER	• Vegetarian Sausages with Tomato and Herb Mash (page 97). • 100–200 g (3½–7 oz) of natural low-fat yogurt mixed with 2 teaspoons of honeycomb and a little finely chopped fresh root ginger.	• Flageolet and Mushroom Savoury (page 100). • Brussels sprouts. • 1 slice of wholemeal toast. • Grilled Pears with Oatmeal and Raspberry Cream (page 104).	•Herb Omelette (page 85). • Small baked potato. • Salad of celery, apple and lettuce. • Lemon jelly made with 300 ml (½ pint) water, served with a small can of mandarins.

DAY 4 & DAY 11	DAY 5 & DAY 12	DAY 6 & DAY 13	DAY 7 & DAY 14
• One of the three breakfast options available (page 47).	• One of the three breakfast options available (page 47).	• One of the three breakfast options available (page 47).	• One of the three breakfast options available (page 47).
• Courgette Stuffed Mushrooms (page 84). • 1 slice of toasted sourdough bread. • Tomato and Spring Onion Salad (page 73). • 125–175 g (4–6 oz) of strawberries.	• Warm Bean Salad with Fresh Herbs (page 78). • 1 thick slice of wholemeal bread. • 75–125 g (3–4 oz) raspberries drizzled with a little clear honey, if liked.	• Slimmers' Coleslaw (page 81). • 1 slice of sourdough or barley bread. • 100–200 g (3½–7 oz) yogurt, either natural or vanilla-flavoured.	• Bean Sprouts with Soy and Ginger (page 85). • 1 hunk of soft wholemeal bread or 2–3 tablespoons boiled brown rice. • 75–125 g (3–4 oz) canned fruit in natural juice.
• Tomato and Courgette Bake (page 98). • Chicory, Orange and Black Olive Salad (page 75). • 100–200 g (3½–7 oz) of low-fat fruit yogurt, with fresh chopped fruit.	• Stuffed Tomatoes (page 81). • Artichoke, Endive and Green Herb Salad (page 76) or Chinese cabbage sliced and gently cooked with 1 garlic clove in a little vegetable stock. • Arabian Apricots (page 106).	• Steamed Vegetables with Guacamole Topping (page 99). • 1 slice of melon topped with a spoon chilled low-fat fromage frais, plus 1 dessertspoon of melon liqueur (optional) poured over just before serving.	• Sautéed Artichokes with Brazil Nuts (page 99). • Steamed baby courgettes and freshly cooked and chopped spring greens. • Traditional Baked Apple (page 103).

Chicken Antipasto

You can roast your own red pepper if you prefer, but peppers bottled in olive oil are much more convenient for quick sandwiches. However, do make sure you drain away the oil in which they have been preserved.

Serves 1

3–4 strips of antipasto red pepper in olive oil
2 tablespoons low-fat fromage frais
2–3 basil sprigs, torn into pieces (optional)
2 slices of pumpernickel bread
75 g (3 oz) cold cooked chicken, very thinly sliced

1 Place the strips of pepper on kitchen paper to drain away the oil in which they were preserved. Meanwhile, mix the fromage frais with the basil, if using, and spread the mixture over the slices of pumpernickel bread.

2 Top the bread with the chicken and the strips of red pepper.

Toasted Gammon Salad Sandwich

You don't need any low-fat butter replacement in this – or indeed many other – sandwiches.

Serves 2

2 thin slices of gammon, trimmed of fat
4 slices of wholemeal and poppy seed bread
prepared English mustard, to taste
2 thin slices of reduced-fat Swiss cheese (such as Emmental or Gruyère)
4 tablespoons mixed chopped salad vegetables (such as alfalfa, cherry tomatoes, unpeeled cucumber)

1 Lay a slice of gammon on top of each of two slices of bread, spread with mustard and top with the Swiss cheese.

2 Place under a preheated grill until the cheese bubbles, then top each with the salad vegetables and the second slice of bread. The bread will soak up the vegetable and meat juices and some of the melted cheese.

variation

You could replace the strips of red pepper with other antipasto vegetables bottled in olive oil, such as mushrooms or artichoke hearts. Make sure they are well drained.

Jerusalem Artichoke Soup

*This delectable soup is equally tasty
served hot or chilled. Jerusalem
artichokes are small knobbly tubers
that are very like fresh root ginger
in appearance.*

Serves 3–4

500–625 g (1–1¼ lb) Jerusalem artichokes,
   thinly peeled and sliced
1 onion, thinly sliced
2–3 bay leaves
600 ml (1 pint) Home-made Chicken or
   Vegetable Stock (see page 37) or water
450–600 ml (¾–1 pint) semi-skimmed milk
1–2 tablespoons low-fat crème fraîche
cayenne pepper and chervil sprigs, to garnish

1 Place the sliced Jerusalem artichokes,
onion and bay leaves in a large
saucepan with the stock or water. Bring to
the boil and simmer until the vegetables
are tender.

2 Add about 450 ml (¾ pint) of the milk
– the exact amount depends on the
quantity of starch in the artichokes. Cook
a little longer, then remove the bay leaves
and pour the soup into a food processor or
blender. Blend until smooth, adding a little
of the remaining milk if necessary.

3 To serve, float a little crème fraîche on
the surface of the soup, sprinkle it with
cayenne pepper and garnish with chervil.

Avocado and Prawns on Rye

You hardly need a recipe for this popular open sandwich.

Serves 1

½ large ripe avocado
1–2 teaspoons lemon juice
2 slices of wholemeal rye bread, toasted
  if liked
8–10 cooked peeled prawns
black pepper
freshly grated nutmeg

1 Score the skin of the avocado half
  lengthways and peel it off in two strips.

2 Remove the stone and mash the
  avocado flesh in a bowl with the
lemon juice and black pepper to taste.

3 Pile the avocado on to the rye bread
  or toast. Top with the prawns and a
little grated nutmeg to taste.

Cottage Cheese Salsa on Toast

Serves 1

75–125 g (3–4 oz) low-fat cottage cheese
2–3 spring onions, chopped
3–4 radishes, chopped
1 tablespoon low-calorie, 'no-added sugar'
  tomato salsa
1 slice of light rye bread

1 Combine the cottage cheese with the
  spring onions, radishes and tomato
salsa in a bowl.

2 Toast the rye bread and pile the
  cottage cheese mixture on top to
serve.

Smoked Cod's Roe with Melba Toast

Smoked cod's roe is often used to make taramasalata, and is a delightful treat if you are fond of fish roe and its deeply smoky flavour.

Serves 1

1 slice of wholemeal bread
1–3 tablespoons smoked cod's roe
lemon juice, to sprinkle
small green salad of unpeeled chopped
    cucumber and crisp lettuce leaves, to serve

1 To make the melba toast, toast the slice of bread until golden brown on both sides. Wait for a few seconds until it is cool enough to handle, then place the slice flat on a work surface and, holding it down firmly with one hand, slip a sharp knife blade into the uncooked 'middle' and slice the toast horizontally into two thinner pieces. Halve the slices diagonally.

2 Toast the uncooked sides and serve the toast warm topped with the cod's roe, sprinkled with lemon juice and accompanied by a small green salad.

Tomato and Spring Onion Salad

Serves 1

1 Little Gem lettuce, outer leaves removed
½ sun-dried tomato in oil, thoroughly drained
1–2 tomatoes, sliced
3–4 spring onions, chopped
3–4 walnut halves, chopped
Farmhouse Dressing (see page 80), to taste

1 Slice across the lettuce to give 6–7 round chunks and place in a bowl. Pat the sun-dried tomato dry on kitchen paper. Slice as thinly as possible and add to the bowl with the fresh tomatoes, spring onions and chopped walnut halves.

2 Add a little dressing. Toss the ingredients well and serve.

Fresh Sardine Salad and Citrus Mint Tabbouleh

Serves 1–2

1 lemon
300–350 ml (10–12 fl oz) Home-made
   Chicken or Vegetable Stock (see page 37)
50–75 g (2–3 oz) bulgar wheat
1–2 teaspoons olive oil
1 handful of mint, roughly chopped
2–3 medium/large fresh sardines, about
   50–75 g (2–3 oz) each
flat leaf parsley, to garnish

1 Halve the lemon. Grate the rind and squeeze the juice from one half and set aside. Cut the remaining half into 4 pieces.

2 Bring the stock to the boil in a small pan. Add the bulgar wheat, reduce the heat and simmer, according to packet directions, until just cooked. Drain well, then add 1 teaspoon olive oil, the reserved lemon rind and juice and the fresh mint. Stir well and set aside – add a little more stock if the tabbouleh seems too dry.

3 Meanwhile, prepare the sardines. Scrape off the scales, then remove and discard the heads, fins, tails and intestines. Rinse well under cold running water and pat dry with kitchen paper. Cook the sardines on a barbecue or under a preheated moderate grill and turn when they are sizzling – brush with a very little olive oil or lemon juice, if liked, but the fish normally have sufficient oil to cook without this.

4 When the sardines are cooked through, serve them on top of the tabbouleh accompanied by the wedges of lemon and garnished with flat leaf parsley.

Viva Tomatoes on Toast

Serves 1

1 slice of sourdough bread
low-fat butter replacement, to spread
1 handful of cherry vine tomatoes, halved, or
   1 large vine tomato, sliced
1 tablespoon snipped chives
dash of Worcestershire sauce

1 Toast the slice of sourdough bread on both sides, then spread with the low-fat butter replacement.

2 Place the tomatoes on top of the toast and place under a preheated grill for a few minutes until soft.

3 Sprinkle the tomatoes with snipped chives and a little Worcestershire sauce and serve.

Chicory, Orange and Black Olive Salad

Serves 1

1 head of chicory, outer leaves removed
1 small orange, peeled
4–5 black olives
dash of balsamic vinegar

1 Divide the chicory into leaves and place in a bowl. Slice the orange and add the flesh and the juice to the chicory.

2 Add the olives and a dash of balsamic vinegar. Toss together well and serve.

variation

You can substitute radicchio for the chicory leaves in this salad for a colourful variation.

Artichoke, Endive and Green Herb Salad

Serves 1

2–3 artichoke hearts in oil, drained
5–6 endive leaves, torn
1 handful of herbs (such as basil, tarragon,
    parsley, chervil), chopped
Farmhouse Dressing (see page 80), to taste

1 Combine the vegetables and herbs in
   a bowl. Add the dressing to taste, toss
well and serve.

Satsuma and Watercress Salad

Serves 2

2 handfuls of watercress
4 satsumas, peeled and segmented
4 pickled walnuts, halved or cut into wedges

1 Mix together the watercress and
   satsuma segments in a bowl. Add
the pickled walnuts and serve.

variation

Combine 2 handfuls of watercress with
the segments of 2 oranges and a few
fresh mint leaves for slightly different
fresh flavours.

Radish Rocket Salad

Try either of these two versions of a fiery fat-burning salad, which goes particularly well with chicken and egg dishes.

Serves 2

2 large handfuls of rocket
6–8 Cos lettuce leaves, sliced
10–15 cm (4–6 in) piece of mooli, finely
  sliced, or 12–16 radishes, halved
DRESSING:
4 tablespoons balsamic vinegar
2 teaspoons clear honey

1 Place the rocket, lettuce leaves and mooli or radishes in a salad bowl.

2 Thoroughly combine the balsamic vinegar and honey and pour over the salad ingredients. Toss together well to coat and serve.

variation

Combine 2 large handfuls of watercress with 2 large handfuls of rocket and 12–16 small, halved radishes. Dress the salad with 4 tablespoons freshly squeezed orange juice thoroughly mixed with 2 teaspoons clear honey.

Warm Bean Salad with Fresh Herbs

Make this for a lunch at home or pack it in a box or flask – warm or chilled – to take for a packed lunch or picnic.

Serves 1–2

125 g (4 oz) okra, thickly sliced
1 large garlic clove, crushed
5–6 tablespoons water
3–4 tablespoons canned butter beans, drained and rinsed
3–4 tablespoons canned red kidney beans, drained and rinsed
1 teaspoon lemon or lime juice
1 teaspoon olive oil
1 small handful of fresh herbs (such as parsley, tarragon, chervil, coriander and dill or fennel), chopped
black pepper
1 thick slice of crusty wholemeal bread, to serve

1 Place the okra, garlic and water in a small saucepan. Cover and heat until boiling, then simmer gently for 3–4 minutes until soft. Drain.

2 Meanwhile, heat the butter beans and red kidney beans with the lemon or lime juice over a gentle heat. Strain, then add the okra and garlic with the olive oil, herbs and a little black pepper.

3 Stir gently and serve with a thick slice of crusty wholemeal bread, which you can use to mop up the delicious juices.

variation

You could substitute canned cannellini beans for the butter beans and borlotti beans for the kidney beans.

Green Bean and Egg Salad

You need fine, fresh green beans for this, topped and tailed, and roughly chopped. Alternatively, you can use sugar snap peas, mangetouts or sprue, very fine asparagus which is just as delicious but often less expensive.

Serves 2

250 g (8 oz) green beans, roughly chopped
6–8 cherry tomatoes, halved
2 garlic cloves, finely chopped
2 dessertspoons toasted pine nuts
2 teaspoons olive oil
4 tablespoons balsamic vinegar
2 eggs, hard-boiled and chopped
black pepper
2 slices of corn bread, to serve

1 Cook the beans (or other vegetables) briskly in a saucepan of boiling water for 5–10 minutes, until tender.

2 Drain the vegetables well, then return to the saucepan and add the halved cherry tomatoes, garlic, a little black pepper, the pine nuts, olive oil and balsamic vinegar. Stir gently to combine, add the chopped hard-boiled egg and stir gently again.

3 Serve warm with corn bread.

tip

To toast pine nuts, which brings out their flavour, spread them on a baking sheet and place in a hot oven or under a preheated grill for a few minutes. Keep checking and shaking the baking sheet so that they cook evenly. Watch the pine nuts carefully as they are quick to burn and will then taste bitter.

Smoked Trout and Rainbow Salad

This simple lunch comprises strips of smoked trout on a slice of fresh wholemeal barley bread, with a little Rainbow Salad.

Serves 1

1 slice of wholemeal barley bread
75–125 g (3–4 oz) smoked trout
RAINBOW SALAD:
1 handful of cress or torn green leaves (such as watercress, lettuce, rocket)
1 tomato, chopped
1–2 slices of cooked beetroot
1 heaped tablespoon grated carrot, turnip or parsnip, or sprouted seeds or grains
a few strips of yellow, green and/or red pepper
6–7 radishes
FARMHOUSE DRESSING:
2 tablespoons cider vinegar or unsweetened apple juice
1 teaspoon clear honey or honeycomb
1 dessertspoon chopped mixed herbs (such as parsley, tarragon, chervil, fennel, dill)
salt and pepper

1 Put all the salad ingredients in a bowl and thoroughly mix together.

2 To make the dressing, place all the ingredients in a screw-top jar, season with salt and pepper and shake well to mix. Pour the dressing over the salad and toss well so that the leaves are coated in the dressing.

3 Arrange the dressed salad on the bread. Arrange the strips of trout on top and serve.

Slimmers' Coleslaw

This deliciously juicy coleslaw is packed with antioxidant vitamins and minerals and, unlike most 'dressed' coleslaws, is high in taste while low in calories. Sprouted onion seeds can be bought from well-stocked supermarkets.

Serves 1

¼ small cabbage
1–2 carrots
2 dessertspoons sprouted onion seeds
　or chopped chives
1 tablespoon raisins
1–2 tablespoons balsamic vinegar

1 Finely grate the cabbage and carrots into a large bowl. Add the sprouted onion seeds or chives and the raisins.

2 Add the balsamic vinegar and toss the coleslaw well to mix.

Stuffed Tomatoes

Serves 1

2 large tomatoes
½ small red onion, chopped
1 teaspoon olive oil
2 teaspoons lightly toasted pine nuts (see page 79)
¼ teaspoon ground allspice
1 tablespoon raisins
2–3 tablespoons boiled brown rice
salt and cayenne pepper
low-fat fromage frais, to serve

1 Slice a lid off each of the tomatoes and scrape out most of the pulp, leaving the tomato 'shells' intact. Soften the onion in the oil. Add the pine nuts and allspice and cook until the pine nuts are golden. Stir in the tomato pulp, raisins, rice, salt and cayenne. Pack gently back into the tomato shells and replace the lids.

2 Place the stuffed tomatoes in a small ovenproof dish and bake in a preheated oven, 190°C (375°F), Gas 5, for 15–20 minutes until bubbling and tender.

3 Serve very hot with a little chilled fromage frais, dusted with cayenne pepper, spooned over.

Crab Salad

Buy some freshly prepared crab meat from your local fishmonger, or get him to dress whole crabs for you if you are entertaining and serve the meat in the shell. Alternatively, you could buy canned crab meat. Make sure you get some of the dark meat – its robust flavour perfectly offsets the blander, more delicate flavour of the white meat from the claws.

Serves 2

2 tablespoons alfalfa sprouts
2 handfuls of watercress
2 handfuls of lettuce, coarsely chopped
2 tomatoes, quartered
10 cm (4 in) piece of cucumber, left
   unpeeled and chopped
6–8 red, green and/or yellow pepper strips
4–5 spring onions, chopped
175–250 g (6–8 oz) crab meat
DRESSING:
2 tablespoons white wine vinegar
1 teaspoon demerara sugar
2 tablespoons chopped mint

1 Assemble the salad, placing the green leaves (alfalfa, watercress, lettuce), tomato, cucumber, pepper strips and spring onions in a large bowl.

2 To make the dressing, place the vinegar, sugar and mint in a screw-top jar, close and shake well to mix. Pour the dressing over the salad. Toss together well so that the vegetables are coated in the dressing. Arrange the salad on two plates.

3 Make sure the plates are absolutely dry of any surplus water from the salad vegetables, then place a portion of crab meat on each plate to serve.

Truffle Eggs

These are wonderful served for brunch or as a dinner party starter. You need a piece of truffle about the size of an index fingernail per person. Alternatives to the truffle are caviar or, less expensive but delicious, red or black lumpfish roe, smoked cod's roe, finely chopped anchovy fillets, smoked salmon, black olives or fresh chives.

Serves 2

2 eggs
2 small pieces of raw truffle, shaved
2 slices of bread, cut into thin narrow strips

1 Lightly soft-boil the eggs for about 3 minutes – cooked whites with runny yolks are essential for this recipe.

2 Allow the eggs to cool before handling, then cut a 'hat' off the pointed end of each one with a serrated knife. Carefully scrape out all the cooked egg into a bowl. Wash the empty shells and 'hats', flicking off any loose fragments. Wipe dry and set aside. Mix the little pieces of raw truffle with the egg and refill the shells.

3 Serve the eggs with thin narrow strips of your chosen bread, for dipping into the egg mixture.

Wilted Spinach with Eggs and Herb Butter

Serves 1

250–300 g (8–10 oz) fresh baby spinach, chopped
1 tablespoon water
2 eggs
15 g (½ oz) butter
1 teaspoon lemon juice
1 tablespoon chopped herbs (such as chives, chervil, tarragon, dill)
salt and pepper

1 Put the spinach in a saucepan with the water. Cover and cook over a medium heat for 1–2 minutes until the spinach is just wilted. Keep warm.

2 Meanwhile, boil the eggs for about 3 minutes, according to your preference – the aim is to have set whites and runny yolks. Shell the eggs when they are cool enough to handle.

3 Heat the butter with the lemon juice. Remove from the heat and stir in the herbs and a little salt and pepper. Arrange the shelled eggs on the spinach and pour over the herb butter.

variation

You could make this dish with quail's eggs, which are delicious when soft boiled. Use two quail's eggs for every hen's egg and boil for only 2 minutes. Quail's eggs are rather difficult to shell.

Courgette Stuffed Mushrooms

Serves 2

2 very large flat mushrooms
1 garlic clove, crushed
2 teaspoons hot horseradish sauce or finely
    grated fresh horseradish
2 teaspoons lemon juice
75 g (3 oz) walnuts, chopped
1 small courgette, grated
2 teaspoons chopped rosemary
½ small onion, finely chopped
2 teaspoons olive oil
salt and pepper
chervil sprigs, to garnish
salad leaves, to serve

1 Remove and discard the mushroom stalks and place the caps, gill side uppermost, in a shallow ovenproof dish. Combine the garlic, horseradish and lemon juice in a small bowl and season to taste. Spread the mixture evenly over the mushrooms.

2 Combine the walnuts, courgette, rosemary, onion and salt and pepper and spoon the mixture over the mushrooms, packing it down gently.

3 Drizzle the olive oil over the top and bake in a preheated oven, 190°C (375°F), Gas Mark 5, for 25–30 minutes until golden. Serve hot with salad leaves, garnished with chervil.

Bean Sprouts with Soy and Ginger

This is delicious and satisfying, and quick enough to prepare in a very brief lunch hour.

Serves 1

250 g (8 oz) bean sprouts
50–75 g (2–3 oz) canned bamboo shoots or
    water chestnuts, drained and thinly sliced
low-sodium soy sauce
½–1 cm (¼–½ in) piece of fresh root ginger,
    finely chopped
1 tablespoon unsalted peanuts or
    cashew nuts

1 Immerse the bean sprouts in a saucepan of boiling water and return to the boil for 30 seconds until just softened. Add the bamboo shoots or water chestnuts and cook for a few seconds to heat through.

2 Strain very well, return to the pan and add the soy sauce, ginger and nuts. Transfer to a serving bowl.

Herb Omelette

Don't worry too much about the technique – untidy-looking omelettes taste just as nice as neat ones; the important thing is not to burn them.

Serves 1

1 teaspoon low-fat butter replacement
2 medium/large eggs
1 tablespoon cold water
2 tablespoons chopped herbs (such as
    chives, parsley, tarragon)
salt and pepper

1 Heat the fat in a nonstick frying pan or omelette pan over a medium heat.

2 Meanwhile, break the eggs into a clean dry bowl, add the water and salt and pepper and whisk in the herbs with a fork or balloon whisk until the mixture is pale and frothy.

3 When the fat sizzles, pour in the egg mixture and tip the pan so that the egg is spread evenly over the base. As the egg starts to cook around the edges of the pan, scrape the edges of the omelette towards the centre with a spatula to allow the uncooked egg to run underneath.

4 When the omelette looks set, give the pan a good shake to ensure it has not stuck – if it has, run the spatula gently underneath. Fold the omelette over, then ease it out of the pan on to a warm plate and serve.

Herb-Crusted Lamb with Spring Greens

Serves 4

finely grated rind of 1 lemon
1 tablespoon ground almonds
2–3 rosemary sprigs, finely chopped
1 tablespoon finely chopped flat leaf parsley
2 garlic cloves, chopped
2 pieces best end of neck of lamb, 4 or 5
  cutlets on each rack
400 g (13 oz) spring greens
2 tablespoons lemon juice
salt and pepper

1 Combine the lemon rind, almonds, rosemary, parsley, garlic and a little salt and pepper.

2 Wipe the lamb with a damp cloth. Remove the fat, leaving just enough to prevent the meat from drying out. Place the meat in a roasting tin and spread the skinned side with the herb mixture, pressing it on well. Roast the lamb in a preheated oven, 200°C (400°F), Gas Mark 6, for 25 minutes.

3 Test whether the lamb is ready by sticking a skewer into the meat – the juices should run clear (unless you prefer your lamb pink, in which case reduce the cooking time slightly). When cooked, transfer the meat to a warmed plate for a short while before carving into cutlets.

4 Meanwhile, discard the outer leaves of the spring greens and shred the rest finely. Plunge into a large saucepan of boiling water and cook for 1–2 minutes until just tender.

5 Drain well and tip into the roasting tin to absorb the roasting juices. Season lightly. Stir in the lemon juice and serve with the roast lamb.

Mixed Grill

Serves 1

2 tiny lamb cutlets or 1 small lamb chop,
   trimmed of fat
1 slice of lamb's liver, rinsed and dried
2 lamb's kidneys, skinned and cored
2 tomatoes, halved
1 large field mushroom
lemon or lime juice, for brushing

1 Using a pastry brush, thoroughly
moisten all the ingredients with lemon
or lime juice.

2 Place them under a preheated
medium grill and cook the lamb chop
for 7–10 minutes each side (cutlets slightly
less), and the liver and kidneys for 2–3
minutes each side, turning as required.
Grill the tomatoes and mushroom for
about 5 minutes, on one side only. Transfer
to a plate and serve with the lamb chop,
liver and kidneys.

Chicken and Winter Vegetables

Serves 4

1–1.5 kg (2–3 lb) chicken
6–8 cloves
1 large onion, cut into wedges
2–3 carrots, chopped
¼ swede, cut into chunks
2–3 parsnips, cut into chunks
2–3 small turnips, cut into chunks
½ teaspoon dried mixed herbs
2–3 bay leaves
salt and pepper

1 Wipe the chicken inside and out with
a damp cloth.

2 Bruise the heads of the cloves and
push their stalks into the onion
wedges. Put the onion in a large saucepan
with a few pieces of carrot, then place the
chicken on top. Fit all the other vegetable
chunks under and around the chicken,
season well with salt and pepper, add the
herbs and enough water to just cover.

3 Bring to the boil quickly, skim, then
lower the heat, partially cover the pan
and simmer slowly for 2½–3 hours, until
the meat is tender. Top up the water if
needed.

4 Divide the chicken and vegetables
among 4 plates and serve.

Harissa Chicken
with Peppers

This is a quick, attractive and delicious main course for the family or guests. Buying peppers preserved in oil eliminates all that grilling and peeling preparation required for raw ones.

Serves 2

2 baking potatoes
1 teaspoon harissa paste
1 tablespoon water
2 chicken breasts, about 175 g (6 oz) each
2 garlic cloves, finely sliced
6–8 strips of red (or green) pepper
 preserved in oil, rinsed and dried
salt and pepper
1 tablespoon roughly chopped coriander, to
 garnish (optional)
leafy green salad, to serve

1 Thinly slice the potatoes and cook in boiling water for 6–8 minutes until almost tender. Drain and scatter in a small roasting tin. Mix the harissa paste with the water and use to coat the potatoes.

2 Using a sharp knife, cut small slits in the chicken breasts to aid even cooking, and pop a slice of garlic into each one. Place on the potatoes and lay the pepper strips on top of the chicken, together with any little bits of garlic left over. Season lightly with salt and pepper.

3 Bake in a preheated oven, 190°C (375°F), Gas Mark 5, until the chicken is cooked through. Scatter with coriander, if using, and serve with a leafy salad.

Italian Chicken with Pan-Fried Vegetables

Serves 4

300 g (10 oz) dried wholewheat pasta (such as tubes, bows, shells)
1 teaspoon olive oil
4 chicken breasts, about 175 g (6 oz) each, sliced into bite-size pieces
2–3 courgettes, sliced
125 g (4 oz) baby corn cobs, halved
12 black olives, drained
1 large beefsteak tomato, thickly sliced
1 tablespoon chopped parsley
1 tablespoon chopped mint
75 g (3 oz) low-fat cottage cheese
2 tablespoons balsamic vinegar

1 Cook the pasta in a large saucepan of boiling water for 10–15 minutes, or according to packet instructions until *al dente* – soft, but with a little bite.

2 Meanwhile, heat the oil in a large, heavy-based frying pan or sauté pan. Add the chicken and cook for 3–4 minutes. Add the courgettes and corn. Cover and cook gently for 7–10 minutes until tender.

3 Add the olives and slices of tomato, and cook for a further 4–5 minutes.

4 Drain the pasta when cooked and return to the pan. Add the cooked vegetables and chicken, the herbs and then the cottage cheese. Stir gently.

5 Arrange the pasta and chicken on 4 plates. Drizzle with the balsamic vinegar and serve.

Spiced Turkey on a Bed of Potato

Turkey breast provides excellent protein for increasing fat meltdown, and is rich in the amino acid tryptophan. This in turn increases serotonin levels, known to help chase away the blues and possibly to help with fat-burning.

Serves 1

1 potato, peeled and cut into chunks
1 teaspoon wholegrain mustard
1 teaspoon ground paprika
1 teaspoon cumin seeds
1 teaspoon lime juice
1 tablespoon water
175–250 g (6–8 oz) turkey breast, thinly sliced

1 Cook the potato in boiling water until tender and cooked through.

2 Meanwhile, combine the mustard, paprika, cumin, lime juice and water. Pour the mixture over the turkey slices in a small pan and cook gently for about 15 minutes until the meat is tender and cooked through.

3 Drain the potato, then sieve it on to a warmed plate. Top with the turkey and its cooking juices.

Prawns in Brandy Cream Sauce

Brandy is traditional for this recipe, but whisky works just as well.

Serves 2

2 tomatoes
2 teaspoons olive oil
2 spring onions, chopped
10–12 cooked peeled tiger prawns
2 tablespoons fresh or frozen peas
2 teaspoons capers, rinsed
2 tablespoons low-fat crème fraîche
2 dessertspoons brandy
black pepper
chervil sprigs, to garnish
4–6 tablespoons boiled brown rice, to serve

1 Place the tomatoes in a bowl and pour over boiling water to cover. Leave for 1–2 minutes, then drain, cut a cross at the stem end of each tomato and peel off the skins. Chop the flesh and set aside.

2 Heat the oil in a frying pan, add the spring onions and prawns and cook for 3 minutes. Add the tomatoes, peas and capers and stir in the crème fraîche with a good grinding of black pepper and the brandy. Stir to mix thoroughly and serve immediately on a bed of warm brown rice, garnished with chervil.

tip

You can make this dish almost as quickly with raw tiger prawns. Simply cook them until they turn pink. Always defrost frozen prawns thoroughly before use.

Salmon with Lemon, Parsley and Tarragon

Serves 2

2 thick salmon steaks, about 175 g (6 oz) each
grated rind and juice of 1 lemon
2 teaspoons olive oil
2 tablespoons chopped parsley
2 tablespoons chopped tarragon
black pepper

1 Brush the salmon on both sides with a little lemon juice and cook gently under a preheated medium grill for 3–4 minutes each side until cooked through.

2 Meanwhile, heat the olive oil with the remaining lemon juice and rind, then add the chopped herbs and the cooking juices from the grill pan. Season with pepper. Mix thoroughly and serve the salmon with the herby lemon oil mixture drizzled over it.

Pasta with Smoked Salmon and Asparagus

Serves 2

125–175 g (4–6 oz) dried wholewheat spaghetti or other pasta
150 g (5 oz) asparagus tips
175 g (6 oz) smoked salmon, cut into pieces
4 heaped tablespoons low-fat fromage frais or crème fraîche
2 tablespoons chopped tarragon, dill or parsley
freshly grated nutmeg, to taste

1 Cook the pasta in a large saucepan of boiling water until tender. Drain and return to the pan. Meanwhile, cook the asparagus tips in a frying pan containing 1 cm (½ in) boiling water for 2 minutes until just tender. Drain.

2 Add the smoked salmon, fromage frais or crème fraîche, asparagus tips, herbs and a little grated nutmeg to taste to the pasta. Mix thoroughly before serving.

93

Sautéed Monkfish with Green Gem Salad

Peeling the shelled broad beans to reveal the inner 'green gems' is slightly laborious, but well worth the effort. You can use canned or frozen broad beans instead of fresh, or substitute fresh or frozen garden peas if you prefer, although the flavour isn't the same.

Serves 2

125–250 g (4–8 oz) shelled broad beans
2 teaspoons olive oil
6-8 spring onions, chopped
250–375 g (8–12 oz) monkfish, cut into large chunks
2–4 dill or basil sprigs, roughly chopped
1 Little Gem lettuce or the inner leaves of ½ Cos lettuce, coarsely chopped
2 handfuls of watercress or alfalfa sprouts
½ green pepper, cored, deseeded and sliced lengthways
4–6 slices of cucumber, unpeeled
6–8 tablespoons Farmhouse Dressing (see page 80)

1 Cook the broad beans in a large saucepan of boiling water for about 5 minutes until tender. Drain, reserving the cooking liquid, and set aside to cool.

2 Meanwhile, heat the olive oil in a frying pan, add the spring onions and cook until softened.

3 Add the monkfish to the pan and turn to coat all over with the oil. Add the basil or dill, then cover and cook over a very low heat until the fish turns opaque and flakes easily.

4 Combine the lettuce, watercress or alfalfa, green pepper and cucumber in a bowl. Dress with a little Farmhouse Dressing and keep the salad cool while you peel the beans.

5 When the beans are cool enough to handle, nick the rather tough outer skin of each bean with the tip of a sharp knife, widen slightly, press gently and the bright green, velvety bean will pop out. Add the beans to the salad and arrange on a plate. Gently place the monkfish and spring onions on top, pour over any pan juices and serve.

Seafood Vermicelli with Tomato and Mushroom Sauce

This is a quick and delicious meal, but don't even think of using shellfish bottled in vinegar or brine. Use frozen shelled cockles and mussels if fresh ones are unavailable and allow them to defrost before using.

Serves 3–4

250 g (8 oz) fresh egg or dried wholewheat
   vermicelli
2 teaspoons olive oil
1 onion, finely sliced
1 garlic clove, crushed or finely chopped
175 g (6 oz) oyster mushrooms, torn into
   large pieces
5–6 large tomatoes, chopped or 400 g
   (13 oz) can tomatoes, roughly chopped
125 g (4 oz) freshly cooked shelled cockles
125 g (4 oz) freshly cooked shelled mussels
1 dessertspoon snipped chives
salt and pepper
basil sprigs, to garnish

1 Cook the vermicelli in a large saucepan of boiling water for about 10 minutes or according to packet instructions until *al dente* – soft, but with a little bite.

2 Meanwhile, heat the olive oil in a medium saucepan. Add the onion and garlic and cook over a low heat, stirring occasionally, until softened. Add the mushrooms and tomatoes – with their juice if using canned or with a little boiling water if using fresh – together with the cockles and mussels.

3 Cook for 5–7 minutes over a medium heat, stirring, until cooked through. Add the chives. Stir well and season to taste with salt and pepper.

4 Drain the vermicelli when cooked and arrange on individual plates. Pour the seafood sauce over the top and garnish with basil sprigs.

Whiting Stoker with Green Beans and Cayenne Potato

Buy the freshest fish you can find – any flat white fish can be used, but this method brings out the delicate flavour of whiting very well.

Serves 1

1 whiting fillet, about 175–200 g (6–7 oz)
3–4 tablespoons water
75–125 g (3–4 oz) green beans
2 teaspoons olive oil
lime juice, to taste
1 tablespoon flaked almonds
CAYENNE POTATO:
1 baking potato
a little skimmed milk, to mix
2–3 spring onions, chopped
pinch of cayenne pepper
low-fat butter replacement or fromage frais,
  to serve

1 To make the cayenne potato, wash the potato, pat it dry and score all the way around the middle with a sharp knife. Bake in a preheated oven, 230°C (450°F), Gas Mark 8, for 1 hour or until tender.

2 When the potato is cooked, cut around the score mark and separate the two halves. Scoop out the potato flesh into a bowl and mash with just enough skimmed milk to achieve the consistency you like. Mix in the chopped spring onions and cayenne pepper to taste and pile back into the shells.

3 Place the fish on a large heatproof plate suitable for steaming or for use in a microwave. Pour over the water and cover. To steam the fish, set the plate over a saucepan of boiling water. Cover and steam gently for 6–8 minutes or until cooked. To microwave the fish, cover it and cook on medium power for 2–4 minutes depending on your oven and the thickness of the fish. Check the fish halfway through – it is cooked when the flesh is opaque and flakes easily.

4 Meanwhile, cook the green beans in a saucepan of boiling water for a few minutes until *al dente* – soft, but with a little bite – and place the potato halves under a preheated grill to brown. Drain the beans and mix with the olive oil, lime juice and flaked almonds.

5 Serve the fish with the green beans and potatoes. Eat the beautifully crisp potato skins, spread with some of the low-fat butter replacement or some very cold low-fat fromage frais from your daily allowance and a little more cayenne pepper, if liked.

Vegetarian Sausages with Tomato and Herb Mash

Serves 1

1 large or 2 medium potatoes, peeled and cut
    into chunks
1 teaspoon olive oil
2–3 vegetarian or Quorn sausages
2 tomatoes, thinly sliced
1 large garlic clove, crushed
½ onion, thinly sliced into rings (optional)
dash of Worcestershire or Tabasco sauce
2 teaspoons finely chopped thyme
3–4 tablespoons skimmed milk
black pepper
basil sprigs, to garnish

1 Cook the potato chunks in saucepan of
boiling water for 20 minutes until soft.

2 Meanwhile, heat the olive oil in a
shallow pan and gently cook the
sausages. Remove them from the pan and
keep them warm.

3 Place the tomato slices in the hot pan
with the garlic and onions, if using,
and cook over a medium heat, turning
frequently, for 4–5 minutes until soft.
Season with a dash of Worcestershire
sauce or Tabasco.

4 Drain the potatoes well, then mash
with the thyme and milk and season
with black pepper.

5 Remove the skins from the cooked
tomatoes, then mix the tomatoes and
onions, if using, with the mashed potato.
Season with a little black pepper and
place on a warmed plate with the sausages
arranged on top. Garnish with basil sprigs
and serve.

variation

You can flavour the mash with a variety
of herbs and spices, including garlic,
parsley, chives or saffron.

Tomato and Courgette Bake

Serves 2

200 g (7 oz) small vine tomatoes, halved
2 small courgettes, thinly sliced
2 teaspoons chopped thyme
2 garlic cloves, finely chopped
2 teaspoons olive oil
4 eggs
3 tablespoons semi-skimmed milk
2 tablespoons freshly grated Parmesan
   cheese
salt and pepper
salad leaves, to serve

1 Lightly oil a 900 ml (1½ pint) shallow ovenproof dish or two individual dishes and scatter with the tomatoes, courgettes, thyme and garlic. Season lightly with salt and pepper. Add the oil and toss to mix. Bake in a preheated oven, 200°C (400°F), Gas Mark 6, for 10 minutes.

2 Lightly beat the eggs with the milk and a little salt and pepper and pour the mixture over the vegetables. Sprinkle with the cheese and bake for a further 30 minutes until golden and lightly set. Serve with salad leaves.

Steamed Vegetables with Guacamole Topping

Serves 1

2–3 carrots, sliced lengthways
1 handful of broccoli florets
1 handful of cauliflower florets
½ large or 1 medium leek, sliced into rings
125 g (4 oz) fresh green beans
½ avocado, mashed
1 spring onion, finely chopped
1 teaspoon curry paste
1 teaspoon chopped coriander
2 cherry tomatoes, chopped
garlic salt and pepper

1 Place the carrots, broccoli, cauliflower, leek and green beans in a metal steamer or sieve and set it over a saucepan of boiling water for 10–12 minutes until the vegetables are crisp to the bite but not too soft. Alternatively, cook the vegetables in an electric steamer.

2 Meanwhile, spoon the avocado flesh into a bowl and mix with the spring onion, curry paste, coriander, tomatoes and a little garlic salt and pepper, using a fork.

3 Drain the vegetables when cooked and arrange on a plate. Top with the guacamole and serve.

Sautéed Artichokes with Brazil Nuts

Substitute a little vegetable broth if you do not have a juicer with which to make fresh carrot juice.

Serves 2

1 onion, thinly sliced
1 teaspoon olive oil
8–10 canned artichoke hearts in brine, rinsed and halved
300 ml (½ pint) freshly prepared carrot juice
grated rind and juice of 1 lime
175 g (6 oz) Brazil nuts, chopped
1 tablespoon snipped chives
pinch of freshly grated nutmeg
salt and pepper
steamed green vegetables, to serve

1 Gently fry the onion in the olive oil in a frying pan until soft but not brown.

2 Add the halved artichoke hearts and carrot juice. Stir in the lime rind and juice, Brazil nuts, chives, nutmeg and salt and pepper until well blended and piping hot. Serve immediately with steamed green vegetables.

Fruit Fanfare

Serves 1

1 large slice of melon
1 small bunch of seedless grapes (about
   15–20)
5–6 cherries, pitted
1 mandarin orange, segmented
3–4 mint sprigs, chopped
5 mm (¼ in) piece of fresh root ginger,
   finely chopped

1 Chop the melon flesh and place in a
   small bowl. Add the remaining fruit,
the mint leaves and the ginger. Mix well.

2 Chill thoroughly in the refrigerator
   before serving.

Walnut and Honey Yogurt

*You should be able to buy honeycomb
from a number of places, such as
healthfood stores, delicatessens or
farm shops selling local produce.*

Serves 1

1 dessertspoon honeycomb
100–200 g (3½–7 oz) low-fat, thick
   natural yogurt
6–7 walnut halves

1 Cut the honeycomb into pieces to
   release the liquid honey from the cells.

2 Stir the honey into the yogurt with the
   walnut halves and serve chilled.

Persimmon Cream

Persimmons are a full red/orange colour when ripe, and feel very soft when squeezed.

Serves 1

1 large persimmon
1 tablespoon low-fat crème fraîche

1 Slice the top off the fruit. Scoop out the fleshy contents into a small bowl and reserve the skin. Add the crème fraîche to the bowl and mix well.

2 Return the persimmon cream to the reserved skin, working carefully because the fleshy 'walls' of the ripe fruit are delicate and easily ruptured. Serve.

Traditional Baked Apple

Serves 1

1 large dessert apple
2–3 cloves
2 tablespoons mixed raisins and sultanas
1 teaspoon clear honey
pinch of ground cinnamon
1 teaspoon brandy (optional)
low-fat natural yogurt, fromage frais or soya
  milk yogurt, to serve

1 Remove and discard the core of the apple using an apple corer. Score around the middle of the apple with a sharp knife to allow it to swell without bursting. Bruise the cloves and push them into the apple.

2 Place the apple in an ovenproof dish or small roasting tin. Mix together the dried fruit, honey and cinnamon and spoon the mixture into the hollowed centre of the apple. Add a teaspoon of brandy if liked. Pour a little hot water into the dish or roasting tin.

3 Cook in a preheated oven, 200°C (400°F), Gas Mark 6, for 45–60 minutes, until very soft. After about 20 minutes baste the apple with the juices in the dish.

4 Serve hot, warm or chilled with a little low-fat natural yogurt, fromage frais or soya milk yogurt.

Grilled Pears with Oatmeal and Raspberry Cream

Serves 1

1 pear, halved
1 teaspoon unrefined icing sugar
2 teaspoons low-fat thick Greek yogurt
2 teaspoons medium oatmeal, toasted
2 dessertspoons raspberries
mint sprigs, to decorate

1 Scoop the cores from the pear halves and place the fruit in a flameproof dish. Dust with the icing sugar and cook under a preheated moderate grill for 3–4 minutes until beginning to colour.

2 Tip the yogurt into a small bowl. Fold in the oatmeal and raspberries, then spoon the mixture into the centres of the pear halves and serve decorated with mint sprigs and a few raspberries.

Warm Pineapple Gratin

Serves 2

4 thick slices of pineapple
2 teaspoons pineapple liqueur or brandy (optional)
½ teaspoon vanilla extract
4 tablespoons low-fat fromage frais, chilled
2 teaspoons light muscovado sugar

1 Place the slices of pineapple in a shallow flameproof dish and sprinkle with the pineapple liqueur or brandy, if using.

2 Stir the vanilla into the fromage frais and spoon the mixture over the pineapple. Sprinkle the sugar over the top, then place under a preheated grill for a few minutes until the sugar is bubbling. Serve at once.

Lychees with Almond Junket

Junket is an old English country dish and was part of staple fare long before the advent of yogurt. Rennet, available from healthfood stores, is produced from an enzyme found in a cow's stomach and is used for creating curds (milk solids) and whey (the watery part). Warming the milk above blood temperature (98.4°F/37°C) will inactivate the rennet and your junket will not set.

Serves 2–3

600 ml (1 pint) semi-skimmed milk
1 dessertspoon demerara sugar
1–2 teaspoons rennet
2–3 drops of real almond essence
250 g (8 oz) can lychees in juice or 250 g
   (8 oz) fresh lychees, skinned and poached
   in a little water

1 Gently heat the semi-skimmed milk in a pan to blood temperature. (When you dip your little finger into the milk, it registers neither hot nor cold.)

2 Pour the warmed milk into a dish and stir in the demerara sugar, rennet and almond essence. Cover and leave to set, then chill in the refrigerator.

3 When the junket is set, cut criss-crosses through it with a knife, and place the lychees between the resulting diamond-shaped curds, together with a little juice.

variation

Vegetarian rennet, derived from plant sources or manufactured synthetically, is also available.

Arabian Apricots

Select really soft, tender apricots for this recipe. Tahini is a thick, oily, light brown paste of crushed toasted sesame seeds. It often separates on standing in the jar, so stir it well before using.

Serves 1

6 presoaked dried apricots
3 teaspoons tahini
ground cinnamon, to taste
6 freshly blanched almonds
1 teaspoon unrefined icing sugar

1 Cut a slit in each apricot. Insert ½ teaspoon tahini mixed with a pinch of ground cinnamon and one blanched almond into each apricot.

2 Reshape the apricots. Sprinkle with icing sugar and set aside for dessert.

Redcurrant Glass Ceiling

Here, demerara sugar is sprinkled over wet redcurrants and left overnight. The sugar and redcurrant juices mingle to form a delicious 'glassy' crust.

Serves 2

250–300 g (8–10 oz) redcurrants
2–4 dessertspoons demerara sugar
½ teaspoon ground cinnamon

1 Remove the redcurrants from their stalks and wash. Place in a dish while still wet.

2 Combine the demerara sugar with the ground cinnamon, then sprinkle the mixture over the redcurrants. Place the dish in the refrigerator and leave to form a glassy crust overnight.

Apple and Blueberry Crumble

Serves 2

2 crisp dessert apples
2 tablespoons water
1 small handful of blueberries
25 g (1 oz) porridge oats
2 teaspoons light olive oil
1 tablespoon light muscovado sugar
25 g (1 oz) sultanas or raisins
mint sprigs, to decorate
low-fat Greek yogurt, to serve

1 Peel, core and slice the apples. Put in a small pan with the water. Cover and cook gently until the apples have softened. Stir in three-quarters of the blueberries and remove from the heat. Allow to cool.

2 Meanwhile, put the oats, oil, sugar and dried fruit in a frying pan and cook, stirring constantly, until the oats are golden. Allow to cool.

3 Divide the apple mixture between two dessert glasses and spoon the oat mixture on top. Top with a spoonful of yogurt, the remaining blueberries and mint sprigs to decorate.

108

6 Just to Remind You. . .

why other diets fail

Fad diets work (briefly) for a number of reasons, not the least being the 'short sharp shock' they deliver to your digestive, glandular, muscular and other systems. The body does react with weight loss when you feed it nothing but, say, lettuce, tomato and cottage cheese, or steak, grapes and spinach, after experiencing months or years of making poor food choices for weight control.

This weight loss does tend to consist mainly of water because such drastic eating plans rely on the metabolic shock of an enormously reduced calorie intake without the help of fat-burner foods. It is also next to impossible to sustain such diets for any length of time, because sooner or later our taste buds will revolt at the fare they are being offered. Never – we feel – will we be able to look a carton of low-fat cottage cheese or a lettuce leaf in the face again. Boredom is the arch enemy of the serious weight-loser, and one you need never do battle with again when you embark upon the Fat-burner Foods Weight Loss Programme.

people in a hurry

remember less than they think – and hope – they will. It is undoubtedly boring and tiring to read or hear the same old thing time and time again when you are so stressed and busy that you hardly have a moment to yourself to breathe freely.

But habits, especially unhealthy ones, become entrenched simply because we repeat them over and over again. It is important, therefore, to remember the importance of alternating your two 14-day plans – the Fat-burner Foods Rapid Fat Loss Plan and the Fat-burner Foods Stabilizer Plan.

two weeks on/two weeks off

So, to remind you, here's what you have to do:

1 Follow the FBF Rapid Fat Loss Plan in Chapter 3 for exactly two weeks. (Week 2 is a repetition of Week 1.) Weigh yourself first thing every morning, without clothes, after going to the toilet. Record your weight on the charts provided on pages 122–123.

2 Follow this immediately – don't be tempted to have a complete rest for a few days – with two weeks on one of the four FBF Stabilizer Plans. (Again, Week 2 is a repetition of Week 1.)

3 If you have more fat to burn, back you go on the Rapid Fat Loss Plan.

4 After two weeks, come off the Rapid Fat Loss Plan again, and on to your choice of FBF Stabilizer Plan.

5 Continue in this way following the Programme exactly, that is two weeks on the Rapid Fat Loss Plan, followed by two weeks on your choice of Stabilizer Plan, as often as you need, until you reach 1–1.5 kg (2–3 lb) below your goal weight, or 0.5 kg (1 lb) if you had only a few pounds to lose to start off with.

6 Continue to check your weight daily or, at the very least, weekly. If your weight should ever climb to 0.5–1 kg (1–2 lb) above your target weight, go back on the FBF Weight Loss Programme until you return to your earlier desirable weight. It really is that simple.

boosting the fat-burning fires

To help yourself achieve your personal goal, continue to vary your diet as much as possible, utilizing the fullest possible range of fat-burner foods and tips. Never go hungry – there's no need – and never despair. Many of the people who have lost all the fat they wanted on the Fat-burner Foods Weight Loss Programme had been overweight for ten, twenty, and in some cases for over thirty years.

There are various ways to boost your fat-burning fires on the Fat-burner Foods Weight Loss Programme, such as drinking plenty of water and eating breakfast. All of these helpful tips are just as useful after you have reached your target weight, when you are determined to remain slim, active and healthy. In addition, don't even think about missing meals or cutting back too drastically on fat – either way, your metabolism will feel threatened by starvation, and drop right down to protect you. Your calorie-burning power therefore tumbles.

Too much fat, on the other hand, may make you eat too much and cancel some of the fat-melting effects of your eating plan. Very overweight people tend to have their appetites stimulated by a high-fat meal, while lean people do not. It is thought that, probably owing to insulin resistance (see page 22), a high fat intake makes an overweight person hungry for more fat-laden foods.

One important part of the FBF Weight Loss Programme is 'grazing', which means eating frequent small meals and permitted snacks, including low-fat protein foods, such as cottage cheese, chicken and fish. Five to six hours during the day is too long to go empty. Three meals a day will raise the metabolic rate by up to 200 calories per 24 hours and grazing boosts it even higher.

A whole range of nutrients work together to produce energy, particularly B group vitamins. Good choices include whole grains, corn, fish and chicken because they can use up more energy than they supply – this means they are also sources of negative calories.

coffee and tea

Be healthwise about coffee and tea. Both tea and coffee increase the rate of metabolism. Enjoy as much as you want of either or both, unless they give you heartburn or palpitations, or you have a heart condition.

A study of green tea reported in the *European Journal of Clinical Nutrition* in 2000 tested the effects of drinking three different strengths – 2.5 g (⅛ oz) of dried leaves in 150 ml (¼ pint) of water, 5 g (¼ oz) in 300 ml (½ pint), and 7.5 g (⅓ oz) in 450 ml (¾ pint) – in ten healthy adults. A standardized laboratory test was used to measure the capacity of the volunteers' plasma (the liquid part of the bloodstream) to neutralize free radicals, harmful molecular fragments that can cause premature ageing, heart disease and cancer. Blood samples were taken one and two hours after drinking the tea, and the two higher doses of tea were found to increase antioxidant activity by approximately 7 and 12 per cent respectively. This is very good news indeed for general health and it might also indicate that other nutrients which are more directly concerned with the body's energy production were equally active.

exercise

Exercise, too, as everyone is aware, revs up fat-burning (see Chapter 7). According to Ian Marber, author of *The Food Doctor in the City*, it enhances the metabolic rate by multiplying the number of mitochondria in muscle cells (mitochondria are the microscopic power houses within cells which convert glucose into energy). Regular exercise sustained for 25–30 minutes four or five times a week can have a significant effect on fat-burning, raising energy consumption for up to 18 hours afterwards.

Making Your Fat-burner Foods Work

ACTION	EFFECT	TO HELP YOU...
Drink at least 8 glasses of water daily	Avoids dehydration, which reduces metabolic rate by 2–3 per cent. Vary the types of water, such as still mineral water, tap water and specialist spring waters.	Add a slice of lemon or lime, or drink hot water flavoured with a pinch of ground nutmeg or cinnamon or small pieces of chopped fresh root ginger.
Eat breakfast	Raises metabolic rate by between 10 and 25 per cent.	Divide your breakfast into two or three snacks if you really cannot eat shortly after waking, for example drink some fruit juice to start the day, eat low-fat yogurt when you get to work/college and then have an apple at mid-morning.
Avoid crash-dieting	Lowers metabolic rate and also deprives your body of essential nutrients.	The nutritionally sound Rapid Fat Loss Plan is hard-hitting like some crash diets, but also prevents the fall in metabolism that unwise diets can cause.
Spread your fat over the course of a day	When you are very overweight a lot of fat eaten all at once can sharpen the appetite for further fat.	Save the low-fat butter replacement intended for breakfast for your lunchtime bread, and eat low-fat yogurt or cheese in the later part of the day. Avoid cheese last thing if it makes you dream, although calcium-rich foods can actually calm the nerves and help promote sound sleep.
'Graze' instead of eating one or two heavy meals per day with long gaps between	'Grazing' uses up to 200 extra calories over 24 hours – equivalent to just under 25 g (1 oz) fat per 24 hours.	Most meals can be divided into at least two parts. Eat little and often – every 2–3 hours.

ACTION	EFFECT	TO HELP YOU...
Eat negative calorie foods daily	They boost fat-burning by using up more calories than they supply.	Many vegetables and low-GI items are negative calorie foods (see page 27).
Drink tea and coffee (see page 113)	Increases metabolic rate and fat burning.	Avoid too many cups of strong, bitter Mediterranean– or Greek–style black coffee, especially on an empty stomach. It can cause nausea and vomiting.
Eat all the spicy foods you enjoy, often	Spices not only perk up bland foods, they also whizz up your metabolic rate by a hefty 25 per cent. Chilli pepper, cayenne and hot mustard should all hit the spot.	You can add all the spices you like to your Fat-burning Soup and to Stabilizer Plan recipes as well.
Exercise! **IMPORTANT: Consult your doctor before starting an exercise programme if you have a medical condition or any health concerns.**	Increases metabolic rate and fat-burning by multiplying the number of mitochondria in the muscles (cellular power houses converting glucose into energy). Regular exercise sustained for 25–30 minutes four or five times a week fans the fat-burning flames within, for up to 18 hours afterwards. Brisk walking, cycling, dancing and swimming are all safe forms of aerobic exercise (the type that makes you slightly out of breath). Simply becoming more active in your everyday routine is also very beneficial.	Drink a cup of coffee 1 hour before exercising. Caffeine triggers the release of fat into the blood, which the exercise will then burn. Iced coffee is delicious in hot weather or any time you fancy. Skimmed milk makes excellent cappuccino – just invest in a hand-held milk frother. Replace fattening chocolate powder with ground cinnamon or nutmeg sprinkled on your cappuccino instead – many coffee shops will do this if you ask.

▶ Deep breathing

▶ Weight training

▶ Aerobic exercise, plus activity
and energy use chart

7 Lighting the Fire Within

deep breathing

Do deep breathing exercises on waking in the morning, before going to sleep at night and at least once during the day.

Stand easily – or lie down, if you happen to be in bed. Take a deep breath S-L-O-W-L-Y over a count of 5 seconds – use a watch or count 'one-thousand-two-thousand...' at medium speed to check the time. Fill your lungs as full as possible.

Hold your breath for 20 seconds, or for as long as you can without straining yourself, and then breathe out again very slowly to a count of 10. Repeat a total of 15 times.

Through this deep breathing, you will see and feel your abdomen expanding in addition to your chest as you breathe in; you will also feel calmer and more stress free, as well as having increased energy.

weight training

Some authorities claim that this is the best fat-burning exercise on the grounds that the metabolism continues to burn at an increased rate for 24 hours after a 60-minute workout. Such a figure (and those of the exercise types in the chart opposite), can be misleading since we vary so much as individuals. However, weight training does have in its favour the development of greater lean muscle mass with its ability to utilize surplus calories more much efficiently.

It also firms and tones the figure, while combating any muscular wastage that can result from prolonged dieting. Together with aerobic exercise or increased general daily activity, weight training also helps to boost the body's metabolism when the calorie intake is reduced.

aerobic exercise

Aerobic exercise makes you slightly breathless and increases your pulse rate. There are plenty of books and videos on working out safely, but it is safest to check with your doctor before starting aerobic exercise for the first time, especially if you have any health concerns. To obtain maximum fat-burning benefits, you should aim eventually to exercise for about 30–40 minutes at a stretch, three to five times a week.

It's important to choose something you really enjoy, be it horse riding, aqua-aerobics or jazz dance. You can share your new activity with a friend, or join a class with them for mutual support and a good laugh!

Build your new activity gradually into your lifestyle. If you do it five days a week for a fortnight, the chances are that you will go right off it and never do it again. The box on this page gives a guide to some activities, together with the energy they use per hour.

Some of these activities – housework, window and cleaning mowing the lawn– are more work than pleasure. So by simply increasing your overall daily activity you can significantly improve overall fitness and energy levels – even if it has less fat-burning boost than the more demanding stuff. Simple ways to do this include using the stairs instead of lifts or escalators, parking further from your destination and walking the rest of the way, and getting up from your desk every hour for a walk around the office or home.

activity and energy use

ACTIVITY	CALORIES/HOUR
Bowling	250
Cleaning windows	350
Cycling	400
Dancing	300
Football	450
Gardening	250
General housework	190
Golf	250
Horse riding	450
Ironing	250
Jogging	500
Mowing the lawn	400
Running	900
Scrubbing floors	275
Skiing	500
Swimming	500
Walking	250

Desirable Weight Ranges

WOMEN

Height	1.45 m	4 ft 9 in	1.65 m	5 ft 5 in
Small frame	40.82 kg – 43.10 kg	90 lb – 97 lb	51.71 kg – 55.80 kg	114 lb – 123 lb
Medium frame	42.64 kg – 48.08 kg	94 lb – 106 lb	54.43 kg – 61.24 kg	120 lb – 135 lb
Large frame	46.27 kg – 53.52 kg	102 lb – 118 lb	58.51 kg – 66.23 kg	129 lb – 146 lb
Height	1.47 m	4 ft 10 in	1.68 m	5 ft 6 in
Small frame	41.73 kg – 45.36 kg	92 lb – 100 lb	53.52 kg – 57.61 kg	118 lb – 127 lb
Medium frame	43.10 kg – 49.44 kg	97 lb – 109 lb	56.25 kg – 63.05 kg	124 lb – 139 lb
Large frame	47.63 kg – 54.89 kg	105 lb – 121 lb	60.33 kg – 68.04 kg	133 lb – 150 lb
Height	1.50 m	4 ft 11 in	1.70 m	5 ft 7 in
Small frame	43.09 kg – 46.72 kg	95 lb – 103 lb	55.34 kg – 59.42 kg	122 lb – 131 lb
Medium frame	45.36 kg – 50.80 kg	100 lb – 112 lb	58.06 kg – 64.86 kg	128 lb – 143 lb
Large frame	48.99 kg – 56.25 kg	108 lb – 124 lb	62.14 kg – 69.85 kg	137 lb – 154 lb
Height	1.52 m	5 ft	1.72 m	5 ft 8 in
Small frame	44.45 kg – 48.08 kg	98 lb – 106 lb	57.15 kg – 61.69 kg	126 lb – 136 lb
Medium frame	46.72 kg – 52.16 kg	103 lb – 115 lb	59.88 kg – 66.68 kg	132 lb – 147 lb
Large frame	50.35 kg – 57.61 kg	111 lb – 127 lb	63.96 kg – 72.12 kg	141 lb – 159 lb
Height	1.55 m	5 ft 1 in	1.75 m	5 ft 9 in
Small frame	45.81 kg – 49.44 kg	101 lb – 109 lb	58.97 kg – 63.50 kg	130 lb – 140 lb
Medium frame	48.08 kg – 53.53 kg	106 lb – 118 lb	61.69 kg – 68.49 kg	136 lb – 151 lb
Large frame	51.71 kg – 58.97 kg	114 lb – 130 lb	65.77 kg – 74.39 kg	145 lb – 164 lb
Height	1.57 m	5 ft 2 in	1.78 m	5 ft 10 in
Small frame	47.17 kg – 50.80 kg	104 lb – 112 lb	60.33 kg – 65.32 kg	133 lb – 144 lb
Medium frame	49.44 kg – 55.34 kg	109 lb – 122 lb	58.97 kg – 70.31 kg	140 lb – 155 lb
Large frame	53.07 kg – 60.78 kg	117 lb – 134 lb	67.59 kg – 76.66 kg	149 lb – 169 lb
Height	1.60 m	5 ft 3 in	1.80 m	5 ft 11 in
Small frame	48.53 kg – 52.16 kg	107 lb – 115 lb	62.15 kg – 67.14 kg	137 lb – 147 lb
Medium frame	50.80 kg – 57.15 kg	112 lb – 126 lb	60.79 kg – 72.13 kg	147 lb – 159 lb
Large frame	54.89 kg – 62.60 kg	121 lb – 138 lb	69.41 kg – 78.48 kg	153 lb – 173 lb
Height	1.63 m	5 ft 4 in	1.83 m	6 ft
Small frame	49.70 kg – 53.98 kg	110 lb – 119 lb	63.97 kg – 68.96 kg	140 lb – 150 lb
Medium frame	52.62 kg – 59.42 kg	116 lb – 131 lb	62.61 kg – 73.95 kg	150 lb – 162 lb
Large frame	56.70 kg – 64.41 kg	125 lb – 142 lb	71.23 kg – 80.30 kg	156 lb – 176 lb

Figures adapted from those provided by the Metropolitan Life Insurance Company, New York, 1959.

MEN

Height	1.55 m	5 ft 1 in	1.75 m	5 ft 9 in
Small frame	47.63 kg – 51.26 kg	105 lb – 113 lb	60.33 kg – 64.87 kg	133 lb – 143 lb
Medium frame	50.35 kg – 55.34 kg	111 lb – 122 lb	63.05 kg – 69.40 kg	139 lb – 153 lb
Large frame	53.98 kg – 60.78 kg	119 lb – 134 lb	67.13 kg – 75.73 kg	148 lb – 167 lb

Height	1.57 m	5 ft 2 in	1.78 m	5 ft 10 in
Small frame	48.99 kg – 52.62 kg	108 lb – 116 lb	62.14 kg – 66.68 kg	137 lb – 147 lb
Medium frame	51.71 kg – 57.15 kg	114 lb – 126 lb	64.86 kg – 71.67 kg	143 lb – 158 lb
Large frame	55.34 kg – 62.14 kg	122 lb – 137 lb	68.95 kg – 78.02 kg	152 lb – 172 lb

Height	1.60 m	5 ft 3 in	1.80 m	5 ft 11 in
Small frame	50.35 kg – 53.98 kg	111 lb – 119 lb	63.96 kg – 68.49 kg	141 lb – 151 lb
Medium frame	53.07 kg – 58.51 kg	117 lb – 129 lb	66.68 kg – 73.94 kg	147 lb – 163 lb
Large frame	56.70 kg – 63.96 kg	125 lb – 141 lb	71.22 kg – 80.29 kg	157 lb – 177 lb

Height	1.63 m	5 ft 4 in	1.83 m	6 ft
Small frame	51.71 kg – 55.34 kg	114 lb – 122 lb	65.77 kg – 70.31 kg	145 lb – 155 lb
Medium frame	54.43 kg – 59.88 kg	120 lb – 132 lb	68.49 kg – 78.47 kg	151 lb – 173 lb
Large frame	58.06 kg – 65.77 kg	128 lb – 145 lb	75.30 kg – 84.82 kg	166 lb – 187 lb

Height	1.65 m	5 ft 5 in	1.85 m	6 ft 1 in
Small frame	53.07 kg – 57.15 kg	117 lb – 126 lb	67.59 kg – 72.58 kg	149 lb – 160 lb
Medium frame	55.79 kg – 61.69 kg	123 lb – 136 lb	70.31 kg – 78.47 kg	155 lb – 173 lb
Large frame	59.42 kg – 67.59 kg	131 lb – 149 lb	75.30 kg – 84.82 kg	166 lb – 187 lb

Height	1.68 m	5 ft 6 in	1.88 m	6 ft 2 in
Small frame	54.89 kg 58.97 kg	121 lb 130 lb	69.40 kg 74.39 kg	153 lb – 164 lb
Medium frame	57.61 kg – 63.50 kg	127 lb – 140 lb	72.58 kg – 80.74 kg	160 lb – 178 lb
Large frame	61.24 kg – 69.85 kg	135 lb – 154 lb	77.57 kg – 87.09 kg	171 lb – 192 lb

Height	1.70 m	5 ft 7 in	1.90 m	6 ft 3 in
Small frame	56.70 kg – 60.78 kg	125 lb – 134 lb	71.21 kg – 76.21 kg	157 lb – 168 lb
Medium frame	59.42 kg – 65.77 kg	131 lb – 145 lb	74.84 kg – 83.01 kg	165 lb – 183 lb
Large frame	63.50 kg – 72.12 kg	140 lb – 159 lb	79.38 kg – 89.36 kg	175 lb – 197 lb

Height	1.72 m	5 ft 8 in	1.92 m	6 ft 4 in
Small frame	58.51 kg – 62.60 kg	129 lb – 138 lb	73.02 kg – 78.02 kg	161 lb – 172 lb
Medium frame	61.24 kg – 67.59 kg	135 lb – 149 lb	76.65 kg – 84.82 kg	169 lb – 187 lb
Large frame	65.32 kg – 73.94 kg	144 lb – 163 lb	81.19 kg – 91.17 kg	179 lb – 201 lb

Keeping a Record

Weigh yourself at the same time daily, preferably first thing in the morning after going to the toilet. Record your weight in kg or lb on the charts

FORTNIGHT STARTING:

Day	1	2	3	4	5	6	7	Total
Week 1								
Week 2								
					Total weight loss			

FORTNIGHT STARTING:

Day	1	2	3	4	5	6	7	Total
Week 1								
Week 2								
					Total weight loss			

FORTNIGHT STARTING:

Day	1	2	3	4	5	6	7	Total
Week 1								
Week 2								
					Total weight loss			

provided below. Record your weight loss at the end of each week and the total weight loss at the end of the fortnight. You will feel more inclined to continue with the FBF Weight Loss Programme when you can chart your progress on paper and can see the weight literally falling away.

FORTNIGHT STARTING:

Day	1	2	3	4	5	6	7	Total
Week 1								
Week 2								
						Total weight loss		

FORTNIGHT STARTING:

Day	1	2	3	4	5	6	7	Total
Week 1								
Week 2								
						Total weight loss		

FORTNIGHT STARTING:

Day	1	2	3	4	5	6	7	Total
Week 1								
Week 2								
						Total weight loss		

frequently asked questions

Q I want to lose 3 kg (6¾ lb). How long should I stay on the programme?

A This depends on how quickly you lose the weight. The seven-day FBF Rapid Fat Loss Plan works as a complete nutritional unit, so remain on it for one to two weeks until you have reached your target weight. You can then stabilize your new weight with a further fortnight on the FBF Stabilizer Plan of your choice.

Q What is meant by a week on the FBF Rapid Fat Loss Plan being a complete nutritional unit?

A The FBF Rapid Fat Loss Plan provides some of all the foods that the body needs over a period of seven days – geared to trigger rapid fat loss, of course. You can eat fresh negative calorie vegetables in unlimited quantities every day, certain fruits and fresh fruit juice on Days 1, 3, 4 and 7, dairy products on Day 4, low-GI carbohydrates and protein towards the end of the week, and so on. This is why you should remain on the diet for a whole 7- or 14-day period as described, before going on to the FBF Stabilizer Plan.

Q What if I want to lose only 1–1.75 kg (2–4 lb)?

A You should still complete the seven-day FBF Rapid Fat Loss Plan, even if you reach the target weight after a day or two. Then stabilize your weight loss by completing a fortnight on one of the FBF Stabilizer Plans because this acts as a guide to healthier everyday eating.

Q Supposing I become unwell while following the FBF Weight Loss Programme, what should I do?

A Just what you would normally do – try simple remedies for any symptoms that last for longer than a few hours, and consult your GP about any that persist. You should not be on the programme if you are pregnant or breastfeeding, and should check first with your doctor if you have any long-term medical condition.

Q Are there any side effects of the FBF Rapid Fat Loss Plan to watch out for?

A I am a great believer in mind over matter – many people are highly suggestible and providing them with a list of possible symptoms makes them very likely to experience them. However, the FBF Rapid Fat Loss Plan has a gently detoxing effect, which you can benefit from further by cutting out caffeine and drinking at least eight large (300 ml/½ pint) glasses of water a day. A very few people experience mild headaches, tiredness, irritability, a bad taste in the mouth and bad breath as toxins leave the system. Combat these symptoms with extra rest and relaxation, regular small snacks, skin brushing and a shoulder, neck and scalp massage.

Q I hate water. Can I drink unsweetened fruit juice in its place?

A Sorry, the answer is no. The FBF Rapid Fat Loss Plan is planned meticulously for maximum fat-burning effect, and you should eat and drink exactly what it recommends every day. Try tap water again (the flavour varies according to area), and experiment with the huge range of spring and mineral waters available. You can also drink your water hot, or chilled, on the rocks, with a thick slice of lemon or lime.

Q I've tried lots of diets since having my children but have never been able to lose more than 0.5–1 kg (1–2 lb). Why should I succeed on the FBF Weight Loss Programme?

A You haven't failed in the past – diets fail people, not the other way around. You have every chance of success on the FBF Rapid Fat Loss Plan, since it has been specially designed to burn surplus body fat that other diets have been unable to budge. It achieves this by boosting the body's fat-burning powers, through targeting the possible underlying problem of a slow metabolism.

Q I am getting married in three months' time and want to shed 19 kg (42 lb) quickly so I can buy a smaller wedding dress. Can't I just stay on the FBF Rapid Fat Loss Plan until I reach my goal?

A I do empathize with your reasons for wanting to lose surplus fat quickly, but this is not the way to go about it. Most fit people could probably remain on the FBF Rapid Fat Loss Plan for considerably longer than a fortnight without developing nutritional deficiencies, but the plan's potent fat-busting action limits the intake of many foods normally enjoyed on a healthy diet. Also, two weeks of fat-burning alternating with two weeks of stabilizing has been shown, time and again, to shift fat fastest. You would be better following the plans as outlined, and building some regular fat-burning exercise (see page 119) into your daily schedule. Take daily supplements of multivitamins and minerals, plus 400 micrograms of chromium picolinate, for good measure.

Q I don't eat any dairy products in any form, but get my calcium and magnesium from green leafy vegetables and a supplement (when I remember to take it). What can I do on day 4 of the FBF Rapid Fat Loss Plan where only bananas, skimmed milk (and the soup) are scheduled?

A You sound in danger of developing a calcium deficiency, which can result in weak teeth and bones, and brittle bone disease (osteoporosis) in middle age. If you cannot take, or dislike, dairy products you should be substituting soya-derived milk, cheese, yogurts and so on. I suggest you make this alteration to your diet right away and use a reduced-fat soya milk in the diet to replace the cow's milk. Alternatives to soya milk are 'milks' made from barley, rice and wheat, but check their vitamin and mineral content. In your twenties your body needs around 1000 mg (1 g) of calcium daily, with half this amount of magnesium – more when you are older.

Q I cannot stand vegetables apart from frozen peas. Can I still do the FBF Weight Loss Programme?

A Vegetables are an essential element of the FBF Rapid Fat Loss Plan, and you cannot eat just peas all the time (or substitute fruit). And, unless you eat a great deal of fruit in the normal way, there is a chance that you may become deficient in the vitamins and minerals that vegetables supply. Try steaming mild-flavoured vegetables, such as swede or turnip, green beans, bamboo shoots or bean sprouts (see negative calorie foods list, page 27) or cooking them in a little clear chicken stock skimmed of fat (see page 37). Alternatively, purée the vegetables in a blender with a dash of low-sodium soy sauce or Worcestershire sauce. Farmhouse Dressing (see page 80) drizzled over very fresh, crisp lettuce leaves or cress may tempt your taste buds, especially if you add masses of fresh herbs of your choice. However, an essential part of any successful, maintained fat loss is choosing widely from foods that you actually enjoy and if you truly cannot get to like vegetables, then the FBF Weight Loss Programme is not for you.

125

index

acknowledgements

Octopus Publishing Group Limited/David Jordan front cover right, front cover centre, front cover centre right, 6 bottom right (repeated throughout), 6 bottom left (repeated throughout), 6 bottom centre left (repeated throughout), 6 bottom centre right (repeated throughout), 7 bottom right (repeated throughout), 7 bottom left (repeated throughout), 7 bottom centre (repeated throughout), 7 bottom centre left (repeated throughout), 8 bottom right (repeated throughout), 8 bottom left (repeated throughout), 8 bottom centre (repeated throughout), 8 bottom centre left (repeated throughout), 8 bottom centre right (repeated throughout), 9 bottom left (repeated throughout), 9 bottom centre (repeated throughout), 9 bottom centre left (repeated throughout), 9 bottom centre right (repeated throughout), 29 bottom right, 36, 39, 53, 57, 58, 71, 74, 78, 82, 84, 90, 92, 93, 95, 97, 98, 104, 107/Ian Wallace front cover centre left (repeated throughout), 6 bottom centre (repeated throughout)/Jeremy Hopley front cover left (repeated throughout), 7 bottom centre right (repeated throughout), 9 bottom right (repeated throughout)

Executive Editor: Nicky Hill
Editor: Charlotte Wilson
Index: Alan Thatcher

Executive Art Editor: Geoff Fennell
Designer: Sue Michniewicz

Photographer: Dave Jordan
Food Stylist: Oona van den Berg
Stylist: Clare Hunt

Senior Production Controller: Martin Croshaw